Fundamental Aspects of Complementary Therapies for Health Care Professionals

Nicky Genders

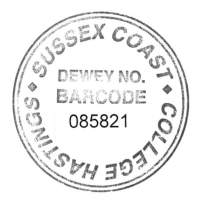
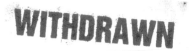
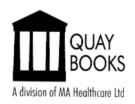

QUAY
BOOKS

A division of MA Healthcare Ltd

For mum and dad and my two children, Amy and Levi, for their unconditional love and unending patience, and to Joanne for her support and unfaltering belief in me.

Nicky Genders

Quay Books Division, MA Healthcare Ltd, St Jude's Church, Dulwich Road, London SE24 0PB

British Library Cataloguing-in-Publication Data
A catalogue record is available for this book

© MA Healthcare Limited 2006
ISBN   685642 269 0

Printed by Gutenberg Press Limited, Gudja Road, Tarxien PLA19, Malta

Contents

Other titles in the Fundamental Aspects of Nursing series include:

Adult Nursing Procedures edited by Penny Tremayne and Sam Parboteeah

Caring for the Acutely Ill Adult edited by Pauline Pratt

Community Nursing edited by John Fowler

Caring for the Person with Dementia by Kirsty Beart

Gynaecology Nursing by Sandra Johnson

Legal, Ethical and Professional Issues in Nursing by Maggie Reeves and Jacquie Orford

Men's Health by Morag Gray

Tissue Viability Nursing by Cheryl Dunford and Bridgit Günnewicht

Palliative Care Nursing by Robert Becker and Richard Gamlin

Women's Heath by Morag Gray

Series Editor: John Fowler

Note: Health care practice and knowledge are constantly changing and developing as new research and treatment, changes in procedures, drugs and equipment become available. The author and publisher have, as far as is possible, taken care to confirm that the information in this book complies with the latest standards of practice and legislation.

Foreword

This introductory book provides an overview of various forms of complementary and alternative medicine (CAM) that have been rising rapidly in popularity among the public in the UK over the past few years. Growing numbers of health professionals in areas such as general practice, nursing and midwifery are now using CAM – together with an increasing range of other therapists with varying degrees of training and experience. Self-help employment of CAM is also rife. Yet knowledge of many aspects of CAM is still quite limited. In this situation, it is vital that health professionals are at least aware of the nature of the different therapies involved and the existing evidence base so that they can make informed judgements for the benefit of patients. This book, as part of the fast-expanding literature base on CAM, will undoubtedly help them in this process, as well as acting as a resource for interested members of the public.

Professor Mike Saks
Chair, Research Council for Complementary Medicine and
Pro Vice Chancellor, University of Lincoln
July 2006

List of contributors

Maggie Brooks DO RGN SMTO is an osteopath registered with the General Osteopathic Council and member of the British Osteopathy Association. She is also a remedial massage therapist, reflexologist and clinical aromatherapist and full member of the Scottish Massage Therapists' Organisation. Maggie lectures at health shows, runs stress management seminars and lectures internationally.

Harriet Di Luzio trained with Farad Davidson in Cambridge with the British School of Natural Medicine and later joined the Guild of Naturopathic Iridologists. She also qualified in reflexology at the Maureen Burgess School at Barnes Hospital, London and qualified in massage and aromatherapy with the Middlesex School of Complementary Medicine. She is a member of the Guild of Complementary Practitioners and a qualified healer.

Claire Jones-Manning RN works as a theatre nurse at the University Hospital Leicester NHS Trust, Leicester.

Edwina McGuire RN practises acupuncture within an NHS pain clinic.

Nikki Murray RMT DIR SMTO is a practising massage therapist and reflexologist at the Attic Fitness Studio, Aberdeen. She trained at the Grampian School of Massage and is a member of the Scottish Massage Therapists Organisation.

Zoe Murrell RN works within rehabilitation mental health services.

Alison Pittendrigh is a UK trained homeopath who founded and runs the Frontline Homeopathy project near Mombasa, Kenya.

Margaret Rakusen BSc PGCE MSTAT is a teacher of the Alexander technique. She runs a private practice in Leeds, West Yorkshire and a training programme for teachers of the Alexander technique. She is also a practitioner of spiritual human yoga.

Sarah Roberts RN practises imagery and relaxation with children in an NHS setting.

Tom Tait is a consultant clinical hypnotherapist.

Catherine Vivian BSc(Chiro) BA is a Bowen therapist who works with children. She co-ordinates the Leicester Children's Bowen Clinic.

Jackie Wiles ex-RGN has completed a course in reiki. She is currently working part-time as a teacher trainer and has recently begun working for the Welsh Assembly as in Inspector of Care Homes.

CHAPTER I

Introduction

What do we mean by complementary and alternative medicine?

A wealth of definitions exists for complementary and alternative therapies, all of which attempt to draw together the multitude of non-orthodox therapies available. The terms alternative and complementary are often used interchangeably to add to the confusion. Alternative therapies are those used as an alternative to orthodox therapy, for example, homeopathic medicine may be used as an alternative to orthodox treatments for specific conditions. Complementary therapies are just that: they complement conventional therapies. However, it is how the therapy is used that determines whether it is alternative or complementary and therefore much of the literature uses both terms and abbreviates them to CAM (complementary and alternative medicine).

If we are to acknowledge the breadth of complementary and alternative therapies the range we must consider is huge. From little known, rarely practised therapies to popular, almost conventional therapies we cannot begin to understand them all. Many therapies have little in the way of an evidence base and are seen as little more than 'quackery' while other therapies are gaining a valid evidence base and are forms of practice acknowledged in health care.

In March 2001 the Secretary of State for Health presented the Government Response to the House of Lords Select Committee on Science and Technology's Report on Complementary and Alternative Medicine (Department of Health, 2001). A key development within this report was the categorization of therapies into sections. These categories have become the outlines for Chapters 3 to 7.

Categorizing these therapies has provided some clarity within health care and the categorization serves to enhance the understanding health care professionals should have of a range of complementary therapies.

Who is involved in CAM practice?

CAM practitioners may have arrived at their practice through a range of routes. Some therapies require years of study, i.e. traditional Chinese medicine, osteopathy and chiropractic, while other therapies may be passed down in one initiation session by a master within that art, i.e. reiki. It is important to recognize this variation in order to acknowledge the range of skills and their perceived importance. For example, for many reiki practitioners the lack of scientific evidence in the practice does not detract from its perceived validity. The practitioner holds faith in the ability of the therapy to heal.

Many nurses, midwives and other health professionals have trained in complementary therapies in addition to their health care qualification but their numbers are difficult to quantify as health care professionals are not necessarily required to disclose or record their CAM qualifications if they are not using them within their practice.

The political response to CAM and the impact on health care professionals

The use of complementary therapies within health care is growing. The role for many health care practitioners, including nurses, midwives and health visitors, in the context of these therapies will be to give information to patients keen to integrate CAM into their care.

So what are the contemporary issues around complementary therapies within health care? As a basis to our understanding of this growth area we need to be aware of the following:

- A large number of patients are using therapies to complement orthodox treatment (around one-third of cancer patients receive complementary therapy treatments and almost half of those who do not receive them would like to do so).
- Around 40% of GP practices in England provide access to CAM for NHS patients (Carter, 2003).
- Nurses, midwives and health visitors are practising complementary therapies both within the NHS and in private practice.
- As the use of CAM grows they are acknowledged within care plans in many areas of health care.

Health care practitioners face a growing agenda around consumer choice. With the increase in the use of complementary therapies nurses, midwives and health visitors need to understand the therapies used by their patients and see complementary therapies as another aspect of patient choice. The following points highlight the considerations for health care professionals around the use of CAM in health care:

- Utilize appropriate 'research' as part of a developing evidence base.
- Ensure that nurses, midwives and health visitors always work within the Code of Professional Conduct (Nursing and Midwifery Council, 2002)
- Ensure local policies/protocols are developed.
- Communicate need with the multidisciplinary team.

However, for many health care professionals integrating complementary therapies into care packages just having a reasonable level of knowledge about the therapies may be limited. The role of the professional bodies in supporting nurses, midwives and other health care professionals to develop their understanding of CAM was acknowledged in the Department of Health Select Committee Report (Department of Health, 2001) with the following statement

'We recommend that the UKCC (now NMC) works with the Royal College of Nursing to make CAM familiarization a part of the undergraduate nursing curriculum and a standard of competency expected of qualified nurses, so that they are aware of the choices that their patients may make.'

And for those nurses working in areas where complementary therapies are currently used, the following statement was added:

'We would also expect nurses specializing in areas where CAM is especially relevant (such as palliative care) to be made aware of any CAM issues particularly pertinent to that speciality during their postgraduate training.'

This recommendation, linked with the clear statement in the Code of Professional Conduct (Nursing and Midwifery Council, 2004) around the use of complementary therapies and the necessity to involve the multidisciplinary team in the decision regarding their use, has led to many developments in the use of complementary therapies in the health care setting. The Nursing and Midwifery Council (2002) states

'You must ensure that the use of complementary or alternative therapies is safe and in the interests of patients and clients. This must be discussed with the team as part of the therapeutic process and the patient or client must consent to their use.'

The acknowledgement of the growth of CAM within health care has led to the acknowledgement of a number of issues around the integration of complementary therapies. These include:

- Knowledge of therapies, including research and regulation.
- Consent.
- Patient information.
- Policy formation.
- Guidelines for professional accountability.

It is envisaged that this book will enhance knowledge of a range of therapies and the evidence base for some of these therapies and encourage thought and debate around the areas of consent, patient information, policy formation and professional accountability.

Understanding the basis on which these therapies now exist for consumers is equally important, after all, for many people these therapies have been a routine way of life for many years.

Challenging Western views on health

Western health care has for centuries had its basis in biomedicine but this was not always the case. In ancient times accepted forms of health care would include the use of herbs and other plant extracts, hands on healing and ritualistic approaches to many health problems. Many healers during this time were women and specific examples include midwives. These women, who were often also healers, were found in many communities (Garratt, 2001). However during the middle ages the rise of Christianity called into question the role of the lay healer with the belief that only God could heal. The following rise of medicine as a male dominated profession with its specialist knowledge and science led to the further oppression of lay healing (Ehrenreich and English, 1973).

The development of the biomedical approach in the West grew as a result of the new found scientific knowledge about the human body. As the medical profession grew the lay healer became more and more marginalized. With the introduction of a free health service in the 1940s the public's desire to utilize scientific orthodox approaches had grown to become the mainstream route to 'health'.

The rise in popularity of CAM over the past few decades has been influenced by a rise in consumer knowledge about health and possible treatment regimes. A lack of faith in the efficacy of some orthodox treatments for chronic health conditions has also led to challenges to the medical model.

Although now not part of the medical approach to health many therapies have existed in a variety of forms over centuries in the UK and Europe with many more arriving to the West from Eastern cultures as travel became more popular. A large proportion of these therapies have their origins dating back over thousands of years.

The role of the health care practitioner

Within the biomedical approach to health, nurses, midwives, health visitors and other health care professionals have played a key role in 'caring' for patients/clients. At times throughout history these professionals may have had the term 'healer' applied to their practices. However, what is caring, and are health professionals in the best position to integrate complementary therapies into their practice? Health professionals, whether they like it or not, have been part of the medicalization of health. The medical model has embraced a scientific basis for knowledge pushing forward boundaries of science and developing our understanding of the human body, health and disease. The adoption of protocols and guidelines for conditions within orthodox medicine has, some believe, moved medicine away from individualized treatment plans and responses to ill health. It has been suggested that it is this lack of an individualized approach that has fueled the rise in numbers of people seeking diagnoses from CAM practitioners. A further suggestion is the nature of holism applied to the individual. A CAM practitioner is likely to take an approach that focuses on the mind, body and spirit of the patient in diagnosis and treatment. This may be in contrast to orthodox symptom control or disease management.

Health care practitioners are directly involved in assessing health care needs, planning treatment/care approaches and evaluating care delivery. In the main this is within a medical model using orthodox treatment regimes. However, two themes are emerging.

1. A growing number of health care practitioners, particularly nurses and midwives, are delivering care where CAM therapies are part of the treatment regime, e.g. palliative care, acupuncture clinics for pain control, and use of TENS (transcutaneous electrical neural stimulation) in midwifery practice.
2. The increase in patient knowledge about, choice of and access to CAM has led to many patients and clients receiving complementary therapies alongside orthodox care.

In the current climate it is therefore imperative that nurses understand the issues surrounding the use of CAM by patients and clients in their care. This may range from having an understanding of the therapies through to wishing to train in a particular therapy in order to integrate it within practice. There are a number of key issues to consider, including the development of an appropriate evidence base to support the use of therapies within health care. Chapter 2 looks at some of the issues around research and the development of an appropriate evidence base.

References

Carter B (2003) Methodological issues and complementary therapies: Researching intangibles? *Complementary Therapies in Nursing and Midwifery* **9**: 133–9.

Department of Health (2001) *Government Response to the House of Lords Select Committee on Science and Technology's report on Complementary and Alternative Medicine*. London: Department of Health.

Ehrenreich B, English D (1973) *Witches, Midwives and Nurses*. New York: Feminist Press at City University of New York.

Garratt RA (2001) The midwife as healer. *Complementary Therapies in Nursing and Midwifery* **7**: 197–201

Nursing and Midwifery Council (2004) *Code of Professional Conduct*. London: Nursing and Midwifery Council.

CHAPTER 2

Developing a research evidence base in CAM

Evidence-based practice

One of the common phrases around in health care today is that of evidence-based practice. Very few would doubt the need for practice to be based on sound evidence but what do we mean by evidence: evidence of cause and effect, evidence of patient satisfaction, evidence of cure? The answer to these questions is all of these and more. Within health care we need to be able to provide the evidence for many aspects of the care we give, not just whether or not a particular treatment works but also how patients feel about the treatment.

Clinical governance within health care has reinforced the importance of evidence-based care with Yvonne Moores, the then Chief Nursing Officer at the Department of Health, stating in 1999 that wherever possible clinical care should be based on sound evidence. The use of electronic resources, National Service Frameworks and organizations such as the National Institute for Clinical Excellence (NICE) were advocated to encourage nurses to seek this evidence base. Where it is difficult to find that evidence Moores suggests, 'Nurses, midwives and health visitors should base their care on consensus opinion of best medical practice.' Moores also suggests that through identifying areas of patient care that need improvement, by actively evaluating nursing contributions and by sharing good practice, the development of an evidence base will be supported.

Evidence-based practice should inform clinical effectiveness, i.e. the extent to which a treatment does what it says it should within available resources. But both evidence-based practice and clinical effectiveness do not rely solely upon available literature and other external evidence they also rely on the clinical judgement of the practitioner.

This combination of external evidence and sound clinical judgement enables the practitioner to develop evidence-based care. McSherry and Haddock (1999) in an article in the *British Journal of Nursing* outline a series of steps that can be taken to assist the development of evidence-based care:

- Step 1: Identify the problem or clinical question from the specific area of practice.

- Step 2: Seek the most relevant evidence from the information available.
- Step 3: Critically appraise that evidence in relation to validity and reliability.
- Step 4: Utilize relevant findings into clinical practice and monitor outcomes, including patient views.

Using these steps, examples of how the evidence for therapies can be explored using this structured approach are illustrated below

Developing an evidence base

Although within health care the randomized controlled trial (RCT) has often been seen as the 'gold standard' in research design this has been because many of the questions we have asked in the past have been about cause and effect: does A cause B? The RCT is probably an appropriate research design in this case but it does depend upon the question being asked. A range of research methods exist and these should be chosen according to the information you want to gain. When gathering evidence ensure that the studies have used the right method for the question being asked. *Table 2.1* gives examples of some questions that may be asked and possible research designs.

Rather than undertaking research studies themselves many practitioners perform literature searches/reviews to gather evidence. This constitutes the second step in McSherry and Haddock's structured approach – identifying the most relevant evidence. This process of search and review of the

Table 2.1: Matching the question to the research design	
Question practitioner may want to ask	Possible research design
Does acupuncture reduce the effects of migraine headaches?	Randomized controlled trial
Is tea tree essential oil effective against head lice?	Laboratory-based study
How many people use acupuncture for pain control and why?	Surveys, interviews, focus groups
Does aromatherapy massage improve the perceived quality of life for patients in palliative care?	Interviews (using self-rating scales), qualitative case studies

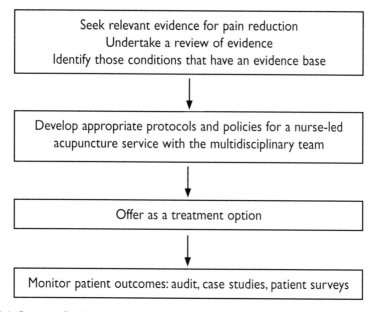

Figure 2.1: Process for the introduction of acupuncture into an outpatient clinic.

literature has over the years been made easier through the use of online databases, search engines and online journals. The initial search may need to be focused to ensure a manageable search can be undertaken. For example, a search for 'massage in nursing' will produce thousands of 'hits' whereas 'the benefits of massage in palliative care' may produce more focused results. Using the most up-to-date literature is also important as new findings are emerging all the time.

The use of a review tool such as the Cochrane Review may also give the practitioner a head start in choosing appropriate literature and studies. Once literature has been gathered a process of filtering must take place to ensure that the evidence is relevant to the question you want to ask.

Once the literature has been filtered, McSherry and Haddock's Step 3 may take place whereby the relevant literature is critically reviewed. This is a further filtering stage but with a more in depth look at the studies. This stage requires an examination of the literature to ensure validity and reliability and to check back against the question to ensure the studies are still generating the evidence required. It is important to review a number of studies to decide whether there is enough evidence to utilize the findings in practice. This then leads to Step 4. Protocols and guidelines may need to be agreed within the multidisciplinary team and policies may need to change to accommodate the introduction of a new treatment option or care intervention. Patient outcomes would also need to be measured alongside patient views.

Figure 2.1 illustrates the process for the introduction of a nurse-led acupuncture service for pain control in a busy outpatient clinic.

The research base in CAM practice

Evidence-based practice is more easily achieved where an existing high quality evidence base exists. Within the area of CAM it has already been acknowledged that in order for therapies to be recognized and integrated into health care a robust evidence base must exist (Department of Health, 2001). In grouping therapies within the Department of Health Select Committee Report the need for a stronger evidence base for many therapies was reinforced.

Ensuring that practice around complementary therapies is evidence based presents many challenges. Three particular challenges include the nature of research and other external evidence, the skills of the CAM practitioner in developing an evidence base and the role of the health care practitioner in using CAM within the health care environment.

Research within the field of complementary and alternative medicine has a history of lack of funding. Rankin Box (2001) quotes a study by Ernst that identified that only around 0.08% of funding for research in the NHS is for complementary therapies. This lack of funding not only has an impact on the types of study possible, but also on their validity and reliability.

There are a range of other barriers to research that may affect projects within the CAM field including attitudes to qualitative studies, ethics committee guidelines and the strength of the orthodox medical community. However, a range of research methods can be utilized within the field of CAM and studies over recent years have become accepted within health care.

It has been suggested by the Department of Health (2001) that CAM practitioners should build an evidence base from research methodologies demonstrating the same rigour as that required for conventional medicine using RCTs and other forms of quantitative research. And for those therapies claiming diagnostic abilities, this must be proved beyond the placebo effect. It does however need to be acknowledged that many of the 'orthodox' approaches used within medicine lack a rigorous research background that has proved them effective beyond the placebo effect.

This has been difficult within the area of CAM as a lack of funding and the complex nature of these therapies has often prevented this type of research being undertaken.

However difficult this is, a number of quantitative studies have been undertaken within the CAM area, including RCTs. Laboratory-based studies often provide very specific evidence of efficacy and many of the studies within the pharmaceutical, cosmetic or food industry have utilized this approach. The effects of essential oils, for example, in a range of cosmetic preparations are common forms of laboratory-based studies undertaken by large resource-rich pharmaceutical companies. These types of studies, however, are very limited within the field of complementary therapies because the complex nature of both the therapies and the practitioner/client relationship often precludes this type of laboratory-based approach.

Qualitative methodology is intended to provide meaning to a question, for example the perceived effect of reflexology on a client with advanced cancer or the experience of massage in patients with Parkinson's disease (Paterson et al, 2005). Qualitative research generally does not set out to prove cause and effect. Many studies in the CAM area utilize this approach to attach meaning to the patient/client experience of a therapy and to its perceived effects. However, these studies are often criticized for their lack of scientific rigour and funding is often difficult to acquire. However, this approach often generates valuable insight into the needs of clients/patients and their perceptions of the complementary therapies being investigated.

For many CAM practitioners research training is limited and, as in any field, the appropriate knowledge and funding will determine the quality of any research study. Nurses may have developed a range of skills within the field of research and may need to consider the research required in the field of CAM in order to support the development of a research base.

Understanding research findings and being able to identify appropriate studies to use as an evidence base to support the integration of CAM into practice are skills that health care professionals need to develop and maintain. A number of specialist journals exist to promote the dissemination of research findings in the area of CAM and health care. One such journal, *Complementary Therapies in Clinical Practice* (previously *Complementary Therapies in Nursing and Midwifery*) published by Elsevier, has a long history of disseminating peer reviewed articles. Specialist journals within each discipline of complementary therapy also exist. However, these may be more difficult to access for health care professionals. A number of databases also produce results for research studies.

Carter (2003) gives an overview of the challenges posed to RCT design. These include:

- Randomization.
- Blinding.
- Matching controls/interventions.
- Shams and placebos.
- Symptom/disease processes.
- Inclusion/exclusion criteria.
- Standardization/protocols.
- Drop out issues.
- Use of sound outcome measures.
- Practitioner–client relationship.
- Influence of practitioner.
- Variability between practitioners.

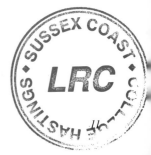

Health care professionals who have concerns regarding research design and the validity of design are recommended to examine Carter's (2003) article describing a number of fundamental challenges to the RCT approach.

Consumer choice may well steer the research agenda as an increasing number of people access CAM. The role of the NHS in supporting this choice has been acknowledged within the Department of Health (2001) Select Committee Report through the recommendation:

'If a therapy does gain a critical mass of evidence to support its efficacy then the NHS and the medical profession should ensure that the public have access to it and its potential benefits.'

It is clear from the Government's response within the Select Committee Report that there is a commitment to acknowledging therapies that have a proven evidence base. The ongoing issue within many aspects of nursing research, not just that around CAM, is the notion of research validity and methodological approaches. The randomized clinical trial may not be the most appropriate form of research methodology for many complementary therapies. Qualitative studies may be more effective but still need to be rigorous in their approach. In general, though funding for research in the area of CAM is limited. A tiny percentage of the budget for research each year is awarded to research into CAM and many authors suggest that change is necessary in order to develop the necessary evidence base around efficacy.

References

Carter B (2003) Methodological issues and complementary therapies: Researching intangibles? *Complementary Therapies in Nursing and Midwifery* **9**: 133–5.

Department of Health (2001) *Government Response to the House of Lords Select Committee on Science and Technology's Report on Complementary and Alternative Medicine*. London: Department of Health.

McSherry R, Haddock J (1999) Evidence-based health care: Its place within clinical governance. *Brit J Nurs* **8**(2): 113–17.

Moores Y (1999) Clinical goverance and nursing. *Prof Nurse* **15**(2): 74–5.

Paterson C, Allen JA, Browning M, Barlow G, Ewings P (2005) A pilot study of therapeutic massage for people with Parkinson's disease: The added value of user involvement. *Complementary Therapies in Clinical Practice* **11**: 161–71.

Rankin Box D (2001) *The Nurses Handbook of Complementary Therapies*. London: Bailliere Tindall.

CHAPTER 3

Therapies in focus:
Osteopathy, chiropractic, homeopathy and acupuncture

Osteopathy

Osteopathic medicine has a history dating back to the 1800s when American doctor Andrew Taylor Still developed the fundamental principles of osteopathic medicine and subsequently opened the first osteopathic medical school. Today osteopathy forms one of the UK Government's 'big five' in complementary and alternative therapies and achieved its status as a regulated profession under the 1993 Osteopaths Act.

What is osteopathy?

Osteopathy is often described as one of the manipulative therapies using both manual and mechanical techniques to redress abnormalities in the bones, joints and muscles. This is thought to re-establish normal functioning to the body's activities. Within osteopathy the view is held that abnormalities in the body's structure and function may lead to much of the pain people suffer. This therapy also works within a holistic framework, acknowledging the body's ability to heal and the link between mind, body and spirit. It has been estimated that over 100 000 people visit an osteopath every week in Britain. A wide range of conditions is treated including low back pain, which, for over half of those seeing an osteopath, is the reason for their visit.

Many patients visiting an osteopath are elderly people and are seeking relief from conditions related to ageing, for example, arthritis. Osteopaths also treat patients for a range of work-related conditions which are often a result of poor posture, poor manual handling or are due to repetitive strain injuries.

A detailed medical history is taken from the patient and diagnosis may include the use of X-rays. An initial examination will focus on the person holistically and not just the presenting condition. Therefore, posture, balance and muscle tone may all be assessed as part of the examination.

Cranial osteopathy

Cranial osteopathy is a specialist form of osteopathy using gentle, subtle techniques to manipulate the cranial bones. Developed in the 1930s this technique has been used for headaches, sinus problems and with babies and children for a variety of conditions.

Training, education and regulation

All osteopaths must be registered with the General Osteopathic Council and it is illegal to describe oneself as an osteopath without registration with this body.

Osteopaths undergo lengthy training on a range of pathways from four to five years on an honours degree programme to postgraduate training for medical practitioners. All programmes are accredited by the General Osteopathic Council. Osteopaths are also, in common with many therapists, required to undertake a programme of continuing professional development.

Osteopathy within health care

An increasing number of osteopaths are working alongside GPs in the primary care arena. A GP may refer a patient to an osteopath for treatment using NHS funding and many private health insurance companies provide cover for treatment by an osteopath. A growing evidence base for this treatment exists particularly around back pain, arthritis and osteopathy in pregnancy.

Case study: Osteopathy
by Maggie Brooks

History
A male patient, aged 25 years, height 192cm, normal weight, presented with pain to the right of the thoracic spine radiating around to the sternum, which he described as very acute at times, particularly when tired. The pain spreads as a band around his chest to the sternum and then slowly fades. His job as a nurse in an intensive care unit involves lifting. He works night shifts at which time he is particularly aware of the pain. The pain eases on rest.

Consultation and history taking gave a picture of a healthy individual who exercised by walking his dog, ate sensibly and was in a good relationship. There was no medical history of note. He had not consulted his doctor about this problem as past experience had shown him that all he would be given is tablets. He came on recommendation of a work colleague.

Onset had been insidious and he could not remember exactly when the pain began but thought he could relate it to lifting someone a week or so previously, although he admitted he was not as aware of his biodynamics while on night duty. The pain was now getting worse and he asked how osteopathy worked.

I explained that I needed to perform an examination to detect what structural imbalances were present and what restrictions there were in movement. Then, once we had identified and isolated the problem, I would work to free the restriction and mobilize to encourage normal movement and the return of balance. I showed him on a model what his problem involved.

He described the pain as lancing and piercing when acute at the level of the costo-transverse joint; it then radiated around to the anterior. He thought it was more painful on inspiration. He reported no numbness or radiation of pain. The pain was definitely worse on pulling movements and when he was tired. It was particularly bad the week I saw him as he was still on night shift. The pain did wear off at times but he was aware of 'something not being right'.

I questioned him about digestive problems in particular, as thoracic lesions often contribute to gastro-intestinal problems. I also asked him if he had any other problems in any other limb(s). I always ask this as pathology in the thoracic spine can also refer pain to the legs, arms, neck or head. I was particularly interested to check if he had problems in shoulder movement, as this is often restricted in thoracic lesions. I also questioned him about any respiratory difficulties because he thought the pain was worse on inspiration. He was not aware of any motor or sensory loss. No allergies or health problems were reported and on discussion of general health, there was no reason not to continue to examine with a view to treating him with osteopathy. The patient agreed with what I suggested and we proceeded to the examination.

I like to offer patients enough time to discuss their problem. I then require them to agree to continue to examination and then to treatment.

Examination
A general observation from all angles was performed and gait was observed. No abnormalities were noted. I checked the pelvic girdle and hips and levels of the shoulders. The right shoulder was lower and the right innominate slightly higher. The whole spine was checked for areas of flattening or abnormal kyphosis. The only noted deviation was around T10–T12 and and there was flattening at T8. (T7 is considered the transitional area where upper limb movements have their axis with lower limb movements.)

I always check the whole body and, if justified, I then examine other areas more specifically. Certainly, had he complained of any other discomfort, e.g. in the sacral area or lumbar spine, I would have examined there as well. I feel very strongly that everything is connected and the dynamics of osteopathy are exciting in that it can help so many diseases.

General observation includes checking for erythema, scar, discoloration, areas of obvious flattening, areas of obvious spasm, or wasting of muscles. Deviations (scoliosis), lumbar lordosis, thoracic kyphosis, evenness in and position of ribcage and musculature are noted.

The patient had nil of note. He had good musculature and some flattening in the thoracic spine with deviation in spinous processes at levels T10–T12 and T8.

Observation and range of motion
General: On flexion, extension, side bending and rotation the only abnormal movement was on lateral flexion which was limited to the right; flattening as mentioned above. Movement of the ribs with breathing showed a slight difference between the right and left sides.

I performed safety checks and used springing movements to check the condition of the spine. Sudden unexplained guarding might have suggested pathology such as a space occupying lesion or even osteomyelitis. This procedure shows the amount of 'play' at each level and thus assists in detecting facet joint lesions. All was in order on examination.

Light palpation showed flashing (erythema) at levels T10 (T10 spinous process is level with transverse process of T11) and T8, otherwise fine. There was no real temperature difference.

Palpation
Palpation was performed on spinous and transverse processes (on the middle and slightly to the side of the spine), over the facet joints (these are synovial joints that need to be kept mobile), and angles of the ribs in inhalation and exhalation applying gentle pressure.

Palpating the spinous and transverse processes for deviations determines whether a rotation lesion is present. Palpating the paraspinal muscles compares consistency and size. The abdominal muscles are also palpated (in flexion), as is rib movement with inhalation and exhalation, and the sides are compared.

Palpation supine: clavicle – no abnormality detected; sternum and sterno-clavicular joint – no abnormality detected; costochrondral joint at rib 8 was tender on the right. (I wanted to exclude Tieze syndrome costo-chrondritis.) Examination of the abdomen included examination of the spleen at the level of ribs 9–11.

Specific examination of the thoracic spine

To examine the thoracic spine the patient is seated and the 2nd and 3rd fingers are placed on the transverse processes (TP) of the suspected lesioned area. The head is dipped forward and back. On forward bending both TP move together. If painful, suspect a straightforward flexion/extension lesion. If one TP moves, that segment has to sidebend to the opposite side, worse in flexion. On backward bending, if one TP moves that segment has to sidebend to the same side, worse in extension. If the TP process is more superficial then rotation is to that side

Specific examination for rib lesions

On testing for an inspiration lesion, lower rib T10 was stuck in inspiration. Expiration lesions only occur in the lower ribs. I placed my hands on the rib cage and asked the patient to breathe in and out deeply. There was a slight difference on the right. T10 stuck in inspiration meant that with inhalation there is a force so when recoil occurs in exhalation, this is not painful. Rib 10 articulates with a single vertebra and as such has a whole facet. I had to consider all the attachments and joints involved. Had I suspected pathology I could have measured inspiration and expiration with a tape measure. This would then serve as a record for future visits, useful for patients with conditions such as emphysema or other chronic lung conditions, which are often helped by osteopathy.

Assessment of the nervous system

There was no loss of sensory or motor function. The patient was alert, communicative, and understood questions. He had good co-ordination and no obvious unsteadiness.

Sympathetic/parasympathetic actuation: The patient was concerned about his problem and obviously finding some movements painful and stressful. I try to leave painful testing to last so as not to stress the patient unduly.

Neurological testing

Kernig's test stretches the spinal cord to reproduce pain. The patient is supine with hands behind head and the head is then flexed onto the chest. Pain may indicate meningeal irritation or irritation of dural covering. Pain on performing the Valsalva manoeuvre (patient bears down as if defecating) may be due to increased thecal pressure. The patient tested negative on this manoeuvre.

T1 interossei: T8/T9 upper abdomen; T9/T10 mid-abdomen; T11/T12 lower abdomen.

L2/L4 quadriceps femoris; L4–S2 hamstrings, L5–S2 Achilles' tendon were all tested. There was no reason to test the cranial nerves as the patient's senses seemed in good working order and he complained of no problems in this area. No abnormalities were discovered.

Treatment plan
The goals of treatment were to ease his pain and to restore mobility in the lesioned vertebrae and rib.

I chose muscle energy techniques to begin to mobilize the thoracic lesion at T10 and T8 and the rib 10 lesion. Muscle energy techniques involve positioning patients in a particular way and then asking them to resist a specific movement. Thus, patients use their own muscles to restore balance.

Once the muscle spasm had eased sufficiently, I utilized a high velocity thrust to mobilize the thoracic and rib lesion. Easing the muscle spasm first ensures that the thrust can be used with less reaction afterwards from inflamed and painful tissues.

Next I performed a high velocity thrust to the costo-transverse joint which 'clicked' and the patient felt the improvement instantly. I used the 'dog' technique, positioning carefully. The patient lies face up with arms crossing the chest and the osteopath lines up the lesioned area underneath.

I then performed a high velocity thrust to the T8 lesion, which had obviously occurred as secondary compensation and it released easily.

I explained to the patient that he might find his complaint got worse before it got better but he told me he felt a 'new man'. I am aware of healing crises, which can be severe in some people. If the pain does become intense I recommend an ice pack (frozen peas) for 10 minutes over the area which should be covered with a thin cloth. This can be repeated twice; I do not advise over-icing. I discussed posture with him and suggested that he make a conscious effort not to continue his holding pattern. In pain, we often adopt postures that become a habit and bad habits are difficult to change. I asked him to take it easy for the rest of the day and explained that I would need to check him again in a week's time as the treatment might need to be repeated as the body became adjusted to the new position.

Second visit: one week later
There had been a great improvement in pain. The patient had suffered a little the day after treatment. However, he felt the pain was coming back and thought he had aggravated it at work again. The pain was not as severe and the T8 lesion had not recurred. I asked him if anything else had happened since I last saw him that I should know about. He said 'no'. I have found that rib lesions that are very resistant to

treatment are linked to emotional problems and talking does help. If the problem is beyond my skills, I refer the patient to a local counsellor.

I re-examined the patient, also checking the pelvis and cervical spine in case there was a contributory factor there. I then performed soft tissue manipulation to prepare the area, particularly the intercostal area, trapezius, rhomboids, scalenes and levator scapulae and mobilized with passive movements and the muscle energy technique used for the rib on the first visit. I then performed a high velocity thrust to the T10 lesion, which was flexed, rotated and sidebent left. I also discussed posture since the patient did tend to stoop because of his height.

Third visit: two weeks later
The patient reported a great improvement and felt fitter in himself. He really saw no reason for this visit so I explained that treating the soft tissues again would most certainly help to ensure that the area did not re-lesion.

On examination, the area of the rib lesion was fine but the thoracic spine at that level was still slightly flexed and rotated left. I mobilized the area with a muscle energy technique and then manipulated with a high velocity thrust. I suggested he return in a month to ensure that all was well. I also suggested coming regularly for a sort of MOT and he told me he would think about it. I discussed the importance of warming up before any activity including lifting patients at work and also doing gentle stretches to the back and also hamstrings, which help to maintain flexibility in the back.

Other conditions suitable for treatment with osteopathy
I have treated successfully the following conditions: migraine, irritable bowel syndrome, asthma, Raynaud's disease, ME, and many painful conditions, such as osteoporosis, arthritis, and autoimmune diseases. If the nerves are compromised at spinal level then the effects are far reaching. Success, I feel, is an improvement in quality of life – this can be more dramatic for some than for others.

Chiropractic

What is chiropractic?

The term chiropractic stems from the Greek words meaning 'by hands'. The therapy began, as did osteopathy, in the US as a response to a lack of faith in orthodox medicine to deal with musculoskeletal problems. Today chiropractors treat a range of conditions including low back pain, sports injuries, headaches and work-related injuries. A patient visiting a chiropractor will receive a full examination which may include X-ray as well as a detailed medical history. Posture will be studied both sitting and standing, and reflexes tested. Muscles are also tested for tension. The aim of the treatment is to restore full (or as full as possible) range of movement to joints. Treatment is given through manipulation of joints and stretching of muscles and may include controlled 'thrusts' which can create a 'popping' sound as gas escapes in the joint.

A MORI poll for the General Chiropractic Council in 2004 highlighted a broad awareness of chiropractic in Britain with over half the survey population knowing what chiropractors do.

There are some similarities between chiropractic and osteopathy. Diagnosis and treatment of disorders of the musculoskeletal system and the impact of this upon general health is a common feature as is the regulation of chiropractors following the Chiropractors Act 1994. The General Chiropractic Council provides a framework for statutory regulation in the UK. However, in the US there had been some reluctance by the medical profession to recognize and acknowledge chiropractic although this has since changed. In the UK a recent survey undertaken by the General Chiropractic Council of its members demonstrated that 76% had had patients referred from GPs in the preceding 6 months, although the numbers of those patients receiving NHS funding for their treatment had dropped (General Chiropractic Council, 2004).

There has been some controversial debate about the risks of stroke due to manipulation of the upper spine. Manipulation of the spine is also performed by physiotherapists, doctors and osteopaths and the *British Medical Journal*'s clinical evidence website puts this risk at between 1 and 3 in 1 million manipulations. Manipulation of this type is thought to be several hundred times safer than the use of non-steroidal anti-inflammatory drugs (Dabbs and Lauretti, 1996).

Training, education and regulation

Training for chiropractors is at batchelor of science level and incorporates medical sciences and skills in diagnosis and referral. Chiropractors are regulated through the General Chiropractic Council and continuing professional development is a key feature of maintaining registration.

Uses within health care

The UK Backpain Exercise and Manipulation (BEAM) trial, a large-scale randomized clinical trial of low back pain treatment, has highlighted the efficacy of manipulative treatments like chiropractic and osteopathy in this condition. The *British Medical Journal* (UK BEAM Trial Team, 2004) reports the findings of this trial and is positive about the benefits of these therapies for specific musculoskeletal problems. The increase in recommendations by GPs for patients to seek the advice of a chiropractor suggests that nurses and other health care practitioners need to be aware of this therapy.

Case study: chiropractic

A female patient aged 87 was referred by her GP with a history of chronic back pain, radiating into the left sacroiliac area, as well as some mid-thoracic pain. She attended the pain clinic at her district general hospital, who did not feel they could help any more. She was advised to do some regular swimming. The referral letter outlined examination findings, including some signs of nerve tension and a tilted pelvis. The patient complained of mid-thoracic pain as well as right low back pain, which radiated into the groin and anterior thigh. The low back pain had troubled her since her 20s but more recently was referring into her groin. The mid-thoracic pain had recurred over the last three or four years. Generally she was worse on prolonged standing and tended to be stiff in the morning.

Examination revealed a tilted pelvis inferior on the left side and associated mild lumber scoliosis concave to the right. Her left shoulder was low with associated mild thoracic erector spinae muscle spasm. The right SLR was painful at 80° and there was some restriction in right hip movement, particularly flexion and abduction. There was a general stiffness throughout her thoracic spine. Lower limb neurology, pulses and abdominal examination appeared normal. A diagnosis of right lumbosacral posterior joint and sacroiliac joint strain was made, with some possible signs of early osteoarthritis of her right hip. She also had stiffness in the costo-vertebral joints of her mid-thoracic spine. A report of the findings was sent to her GP. She was treated on seven occasions with manipulation and exercises.

On her seventh attendance, she said that she was generally much better and was discharged with advice about how to maintain the improvement, including postural and mobility exercises.

(Reproduced with kind permission of the British Chiropractic Association.
www.chiropractic-uk.co.uk)

Homeopathy

What is homeopathy?

From around the 18th century homeopathy has been recognized as a system of medicine that treats 'like with like'. The German doctor Samuel Hahnemann initially introduced the concept when he found that minute amounts of a substance could produce a desirable therapeutic effect without unwanted toxicity. These highly diluted amounts were questioned in many arenas but Hahnemann held on to the view that it was a combination of dilution and succession that released the therapeutic potential from these substances.

In the UK, homeopathy grew from the early 1800s, with London's first homeopathic hospital being set up in 1849. The inclusion of homeopathy as an approved treatment method in the NHS at its inception in 1948 meant that homeopathic hospitals could provide this treatment.

Today homeopathy is accepted and practised in many countries around the world. In the UK the Faculty of Homeopathy (www.trusthomeopathy.org. Accessed 14 December 2005) indicates that sales of homeopathic medicines are rising by approximately 20% a year and that referrals to NHS homeopathic hospitals also continue to rise. However, scientists are still unsure about how homeopathy actually works. Homeopathic remedies come from a variety of sources including plants, vegetables, organic substances, minerals, chemicals, animals and insects. In general the original source is highly diluted to produce a tablet, powder, granules or tincture for ingestion. The potency of the remedy can be varied dependent upon the dilution but the two standard potencies available in the UK are 6C and 30C. Most commonly 6C is used if the symptoms have existed for some time and 30C is used in the acute phase. These standard potencies are available in many health food stores, high street chemists and large supermarket chains. However, a homeopath will provide assessment, advice and a wider range of potencies. Pharmacists and homeopaths will also advise patients to avoid coffee, peppermint or menthol as these are thought to affect the remedies. Many homeopathic preparations also have a lactose base and therefore patients with lactose intolerance or diabetes need to be aware of this.

For someone with a number of conditions the list of symptoms is cross-referenced and checked against other symptoms but only one remedy is used for that condition and not mixed with other remedies.

Homeopathic treatment is based around the precept that the person is more than a collection of the physical parts. A hierarchy of symptoms, both physical and psychological, are considered before a decision about the appropriate remedy is considered. For example, there are a number of remedies identified for hay fever depending upon the presenting symptoms. If the symptoms are of burning, watering eyes, runny nose and a lot of sneezing then euphrasia will be recommended. If symptoms include violent bursts of sneezing, the nose feels blocked and is runny and the throat itches, gelsemium is advised, and if symptoms are better out of doors pulsatilla is recommended.

Training, education and regulation

There are currently two main education pathways to homeopathy. Medically qualified and other statutorily regulated health professionals can train with the Faculty of Homeopathy that regulates the training and practice of this group of professionals and vets who practise homeopathy. For non-medically qualified homeopaths there is at present no single registering body. The Society of Homeopaths is the largest organization for this group and members practise in accordance with a code of ethics and practice and hold professional insurance.

Homeopathy in health care

Around 200 randomized controlled trials have been conducted evaluating homeopathy. The research base has produced some controversial debate around it effectiveness and those supporting homeopathy have argued that the types of conditions used in the research do not reflect routine homeopathic practice. However, controlled trials around rheumatoid arthritis (Gibson et al, 1980) and asthma (Reilly et al, 1994) have all produced significant results compared to placebo groups.

Homeopathy has also been noted as effective against a number of symptoms of multiple sclerosis, notably bladder symptoms, bowel dysfunction, eye symptoms, cramps, spasms and sensory symptoms (Whitmarsh, 2003).

Case studies: Homeopathy
by Angie Jackson

Introduction
The first time you visit a homeopath you may be surprised at the amount of detail required during the case taking. Apart from recording the symptoms of the presenting complaint, the homeopath will enquire about any other ailments, eating habits, sleep patterns, social behaviour, fears, anxieties and general emotions, medical history, any accidents or injuries, and a broad range of other issues. This is all with a view to building up a complete picture of you, taking into account your physical, emotional and psychological aspects. The homeopath's job is to prescribe a homeopathic remedy that most accurately reflects this picture and that will stimulate your system to return to health.

Homeopathic remedies are drawn from all the kingdoms of nature – plants, minerals and some animal substances, such as bee sting (*Apis Mel*). After a highly refining process of succession and dilution in order to make the remedy, the end product, usually in tablet form, is gentle yet potent, safe and effective.

Homeopaths believe that any shock, trauma, or milestone that makes an impact at any time in life will be held somehow in the body unless processed or released. It may be deeply held; it may have been forgotten; it may manifest in a seemingly unrelated way. It does not matter how long ago it happened, sometimes we even hold on to the trauma of birth, but if it is what we call unfinished business, then it is still there for the body to deal with. My experience with homeopathic prescribing is that the remedies can support the process of unlocking that door so that the layers of the past can be released, sometimes consciously, other times not. As these layers melt or peel away, so the original healthy being may begin to be uncovered or revealed, enabling the individual to strive, less encumbered, towards his or her potential. This is one of the aims of the homeopathic process.

Case study 1
by Angie Jackson
A retired businessman in his mid-70s presented with catarrh at the back of his throat, which he had had for many years. He had tried many things and homeopathy was a last resort. He had come reluctantly and on the insistence of his wife. The worst aspect about his catarrh was that he would choke with it, especially when lying down at night. Usually within an hour of going to sleep, around midnight, he chokes and has nightmares at the same time about fighting the Japanese. He feels as if he is choking to death, as if he is going to die. Apart from being very frightening for him, it is also most disturbing for his wife, because he usually ends up on the other side of the room, having flung his bedclothes about the place, shouting at the top of his voice and flailing his limbs around as if in battle.

This has been the case for most of their 50-year marriage, during which time his wife has not had a proper night's sleep. When he wakes in the morning he always feels a sense of relief to be awake and alive, but does not really remember what happened during the night, except that he was fighting the Japanese. His sleep is restless, with tossing and turning, and he rarely sleeps for more than two hours.

He tells me about the war. He was in a prisoner of war camp. 'It was a terrible war, uncivilized. During the night I would lie in my bunk bed wondering if I would be shot in the night or if I would be alive in the morning. I was paralysed in fear.' Apart from this problem he has had a reasonably healthy life. He sometimes get chesty, especially in the cold weather. He also suffers from indigestion with burning, acidity and wind in the digestive tract. Emotionally his main tendency is to worry. He says that he will worry about anything and everything, no matter how small or trivial.

I observe he is meticulously well-dressed, obviously having paid attention to every detail, and that he is very formal and upright in his manner. This aspect of a person is just as important a part of the picture as the medical detail. It helps to provide the shade and the nuance, for differentiation between homeopathic remedies.

It is very clear that this gentleman was deeply affected by his experiences during the war, and in some sense has not been well since, or has not been able to release the fear and the memory from his body.

Here, he is presenting with catarrh in the throat and another aspect of the homeopath's brief is to look behind the presenting symptoms for the underlying cause. It is this underlying cause that needs to be prescribed for, in addition to each person's unique presentation of symptoms.

The prescription in this case was based mainly on a picture of holding long-standing fear and fright in the body, a fear of death around midnight, fear of choking with catarrh in the throat, disturbed, anxious and restless sleep, and a tendency to worry. The homeopathic remedy *Arsenicum Album* is the one that best matches this picture, and it also well suits someone with chestiness in cold weather, burning and acidity in the digestive tract, and who dresses immaculately. Prescribing a remedy is like holding up a mirror to the individual, so that he or she may see what may now be let go of. The philosophy of homeopathy is always of minimum intervention, prescribing the least amount required to stimulate the body to do the work. It is not the remedy which does the work: the body is reminded by the remedy of the work that needs to be done to find the way back to health again.

I prescribed *Arsenicum Album* in a low potency and we met again one month later. He reported that within 48 hours of taking the remedy he experienced deep and restful sleep and can hardly believe it. The nightmares have been less frequent and he no longer feels as if he is choking or fighting the Japanese. The catarrh has gradually decreased and his indigestion is also better than it was. He has realized that his restlessness at night was due to remaining stuck in the idea that to survive at night one had to be alert. Fifty years later that is no longer necessary; he can relax at night now, and, perhaps in consequence, he also appears more relaxed in himself.

This was a very good response to the initial remedy. However, there was still work to be done in order to maintain the improvement so we met on a monthly basis over the next few months, working with the same remedy, until the catarrh had gone. He felt generally better in himself than he had for years, and had reached a point that he had never thought would be possible, namely he sleeps well most nights and feels rested on waking. This is the potential achievable when we release the past. Homeopathic remedies can be a great tool and support in this process.

(Reproduced with kind permission from www.webhealth.co.uk.
Accessed 14 December 2005)

Case study 2
by Alison Pittendrigh

The patient presented to the Frontline Homeopathy project near Mombasa in Kenya with a very sore hand. He was sweating and clearly in agony. The story he told was that he had been arrested because he had lost his ID card (everyone has to carry one in Kenya) and while in prison something had bitten him. It had started as a small itchy spot and within two weeks the flesh across the bridge of his hand had been eaten away and his fingers were beginning to fall off. I could see the tendons and bones behind all the pus and within seconds of removing the old cloth bandage the flies buzzed round us.

I thought that not even homeopathy could fix this. I had heard of a similar story where the person also thought he had been bitten by an insect. I remembered that in that instance the person had enlisted the help of a witchdoctor who had saved the hand and one finger and thumb. I decided the best thing was to give him the bus fare home, where he would be fed and looked after, and some money for a decent meal while he was travelling. I suggested he went to see a witchdoctor in his home area. I also gave him some remedies.

The remedies I chose were:

- *Pyrogenium* 200C (truly bad meat here).
- *Mercurius vivus* 200C (eating away at the tissue).
- *Calcarea sulphurica* 30C (just to keep it all coming).

The remedies were made into one tablet, and I told him to take the tablets as often as he liked. I gave him enough for two a day for about three weeks. I also gave *Syphilinum* 200C (why did it happen to him?) to take weekly for four weeks. I honestly never thought I would see him again and had no real expectation of a good result from the prescription.

Imagine my surprise when he returned some months later and showed me his hand. There was only one small hole just at the base of his third finger which was still producing a small amount of pus. I asked him if he had seen the witchdoctor. No. Had he been to the hospital? No. What, he only took the remedies? Yes. And he went home? Yes. I wondered if he was just saying that so that I might give him some more money but he said he did not want any money.

He told me he had returned to collect a few possessions and he just wanted to thank me, and to show me his hand. He told me that the pain went within a couple of days and over three weeks he watched as his hand began to heal.

He said there was still some pain if he carried heavy items, so I gave him some more *Calcarea sulphurica* and suggested he came back if there was still some residual problem. He has not returned.

(*Reproduced with kind permission from* Homeopathy in Practice)

Acupuncture

Eastern cultures, particularly the Chinese, have been using acupuncture to restore, promote and maintain health for over 2000 years. Since the cultural revolution in China the use of traditional Chinese medicine, of which acupuncture is a part, has increased.

Acupuncture has been recognized within Western health care for some years. It is accepted as a discrete discipline with regulation and there has been a steady increase over the last 35 years in qualified acupuncturists registered with the British Acupuncture Council with over 2500 qualified acupuncturists registered in 2004 (British Acupuncture Council, 2005). Many of those qualified within the UK are medically qualified doctors, physiotherapists and other orthodox health care professionals, demonstrating the degree of acceptance within orthodox medicine.

What is acupuncture?

Acupuncture involves the use of fine, solid needles inserted into certain points on the body just under the skin. These needles are usually left in place for around 20–30 minutes. There are approx 2000 points identified for insertion and within traditional Chinese medicine a central feature of acupuncture is the flow of energy (qi) through the body. Chinese acupuncture identifies 14 meridians or energy channels and the insertion of needles at specific points along these meridians is felt to unblock energy and aid self-healing. In addition to traditional acupuncture the acupuncturist may use techniques such as moxibustion or electro-acupuncture.

Moxibustion involves the burning of herbs on the ends of the needles and electro-acupuncture involves the application of an electrical current to the needles. Auricular acupuncture involves insertion of needles into specific points on the ear. The latter is often used in drug and alcohol addiction to reduce cravings.

Within traditional Chinese medicine acupuncture is a broad-based therapy used in a wide range of conditions with greater focus on the balancing of energy. However, in the West this view is shadowed by the dominant scientific paradigm and attempts to explain acupuncture have included biochemical or bioelectrical explanations.

How does acupuncture work?

The most common theories identified for the efficacy of acupuncture in the West include:

1. The pain gate theory. This theory suggests that pain signals pass through a number of 'gates' moving up the spinal cord to the brain. Pain signals move slowly and the body can generate faster signals in response to particular stimuli (i.e. acupuncture). These faster signals then compete at the pain gates and win – the gate is then closed and pain signals do not pass through.
2. Circulation control and endorphin release. This theory supports the view that stimulation of the acupuncture points triggers the body to release endorphins into the circulation.
3. Neurotransmitter effects. This theory suggests that acupuncture works by influencing the body's electromagnetic fields. The acupuncture points in the body are known to be concentrated in regions of low electrical resistance and the stimulation of these points alters the chemical neurotransmitters in the body.

Training, education and regulation

Training in acupuncture is available through a number of routes. Doctors may train to become acupuncturists at a basic competence level or a further advanced level. Physiotherapists may also train to use acupuncture as part of their practice and register with a body such as the Acupuncture Association of Chartered Physiotherapists which has different categories of membership depending on the length of training in acupuncture that has been undertaken.

Non-medically qualified acupuncturists are represented through the British Acupuncture Council (BAcC) whose members have undertaken at least three years training in acupuncture and Western medical studies. Members of the BAcC have a code of practice and ethical framework to work within and are currently self-regulating although there are proposals to review statutory regulation of acupuncturists.

Acupuncture in health care

In the West acupuncture has mainly been used for pain relief and anaesthesia and in the UK it has been integrated into orthodox medicine in hospitals through pain clinics, and, within primary care, many GPs are qualified to practise Western acupuncture within their practice environment.

The following conditions have been identified in the literature to benefit from the use of acupuncture:

■   Post-operative or pre-natal nausea.
■   Chronic headache.
■   Back pain and sciatica.
■   Chronic pain in a variety of conditions.

- Anaesthesia during surgical procedures.
- Drug and alcohol addiction.

Summary

Acupuncture is being recognized as a discrete area of practice within orthodox medicine. Regulation in the UK is under way to enable practitioners to be recognized on a specific register. Much of the existing research focuses on the Western approach to acupuncture, identifying the efficacy of acupuncture in relation to a range of conditions.

The following case study demonstrates the use of acupuncture within orthodox health care.

Case study: Acupuncture
by Edwina McGuire

Scott, a full-time engineer aged 34 years, married with two young daughters, was referred to the pain clinic by a consultant urologist with a long-standing (10 years) history of left testicular pain. He had been fully investigated by the genitourinary physicians and had had a number of procedures all of which proved to be of no help. Ligation of the varicocele gave some relief for two months after which time it returned. A number of analgesics had been tried without benefit.

Scott attended the pain clinic initially in March 2001 by which time he was low in mood and frustrated with the condition. He did however continue to work full-time and had very little absence through sickness. His attendance at work was important to him.

At the initial meeting Scott described an dull aching pain that built up to a burning sensation over the saddle area and perineum radiating to his coccyx and upper medial aspects of both thighs. The pain was intermittent in nature, with occasional unbearable episodes. He experienced post-micturition pain and pain following sexual intercourse. All of this was now putting a strain on his life and marriage.

He was diagnosed by the pain consultant as having perineal neuralgia but other than this his overall health was good. Scott's management plan was to trial neuralgia medication, amitriptyline and gabapentin. Additionally his plan included neural blockade, as a day case, in the form of caudal epidural plus the use of transcutaneous electrical neural stimulation (TENS) and acupuncture. Medication was commenced but the side effects outweighed any benefits. The caudal epidural gave no improvement and the consultant proceeded to nerve blocks which were again unsuccessful. The TENS machine also did not suit Scott.

Some six months later Scott attended for acupuncture. He was nervous and concerned about where the needles might be placed. Analgesic points colon 4, liver 3 and stomach 44 were used during the session and a week later at his review Scott reported that his pain relief had been excellent. Scott had a course of six treatments and each time pain relief came on the next day and lasted all week.

As these points were all easy for Scott to reach I researched the area of self-acupuncture using the internet to find pain clinics where self-treatment was used and contacted a doctor in a London-based hospital with experience of self-acupuncture with patients. The possibility of this approach was discussed with Scott's consultant and a self-management protocol was devised. This protocol was passed by the hospital risk management committee and discussed and approved by the chronic pain management team. It is vital to choose the right type of patient for this approach. Scott was keen to learn, intelligent, and understood the risks around needles. He was provided with needles, sharps bin instructions, descriptions of the points, plus an anatomical diagram of the points for reference. After three sessions of practice Scott had perfected the technique and was delighted that he now had control over his pain and could administer his treatment when needed. Scott administers his acupuncture every week at his convenience.

Self-acupuncture is now used with 14 other suitable patients at Leicester General Hospital. None of the patients has reported any problems with self-administration and all manage their pain on their own.

References

British Acupuncture Council (2005) From: www.acupuncture.org.uk/content/PractitionerSearch/practition.html (Accessed 14 December 2005).

Dabbs V, Lauretti WJ (1999) A risk assessment of cervical manipulation vs. NSAIDs for the treatment of neck pain. *J Manipulative Physiological Therapy* **19**(3): 220–1.

Gibson RG, Gibson S, MacNeill AD, Watson-Buchanan W (1980) Homeopathic therapy in rheumatoid arthritis: Evaluation by double blind clinical therapeutic trial. *Br J Clin Pharmacol* **9**: 453–9.

Reilly D, Taylor M, Campbell J, Beattie N, McSharry C, Aitchison T, Carter R, Stevenson R (1994) Is evidence for homeopathy reproducible? *Lancet* **344**: 1601–6.

UK BEAM Trial Team (2004) United Kingdom back pain exercise and manipulation (UK BEAM) randomised trial: effectiveness of physical treatments for back pain in primary care. *Br Med J* **329**: 1377

Whitmarsh T (2003) Homeopathy in multiple sclerosis. *Complementary Therapies in Nursing and Midwifery* **9**: 6–9.

Further reading and sources of information

Chiropractic
www.gcc-uk.org

Homeopathy
Geraghty B (1997) *Homeopathy for Midwives*. Edinburgh: Churchill Livingstone.

www.trusthomeopathy.org

www.homeopathy-soh.org

Osteopathy
www.osteopathy.org.uk

Chapter 4

Alternative systems of medicine:
Ayurveda and the diagnostic therapies

Ayurveda

Ayurveda is an ancient medical system that has its origins in India, and is still the most important form of medicine in the Indian subcontinent. Its philosophies are also gaining ground in the West. Classical ayurvedic training is conducted in Sanskrit and most ayurvedic practitioners tend to be orthodox doctors as well.

The word 'ayurveda' comes from Sanskrit and means 'the science of life'. Ayurvedic philosophy suggests that the human lifespan should be around 100 years, and that all those years should be lived in total health, both physical and mental. The ayurvedic practitioner is looking to balance the body and mind, and to find health problems before they occur or arrest them before they do any real harm.

Ayurvedic philosophy is founded on a basic tenet around the five elements – ether, air, fire, water and earth. The elements do not act in isolation, three different combinations of the elements, called tridosha, are what form the basis for diagnosis, treatment, cure and health maintenance in ayurvedic medicine. Each individual's constitution is determined by the state of their parents' doshas at the time of conception; and at birth individuals have the levels of the three doshas that are right for them. Life and all its forces can cause the doshas to become unbalanced which can lead to ill health.

Each of the three doshas has a role to play in the body:

1. *Vatha* is the driving force, it relates mainly to the nervous system and the body's energy centre.
2. *Pitta* is fire, it relates to the metabolism, digestion, enzymes, acid and bile.
3. *Kapha* is related to water in the mucous membranes, phlegm, moisture, fat and lymphatics.

A consultation with an ayurvedic practitioner may vary hugely from one practitioner to another.

The basic diagnosis is known as the three-point diagnosis and involves detailed observation of appearance, examination by touch, and a detailed questionnaire about lifestyle and health. A range of treatments may then be prescribed including herbal preparations and other healing techniques. Massage, exercise, breathing and meditation may also be used as treatments.

Acupressure

Acupressure has been described as simply acupuncture without the needles (Rankin Box, 2001). Firm fingertip pressure is applied to specific points on the body. These points in turn relate to specific organs of the body. Acupressure has been used for a range of conditions but with little research into its efficacy. The most common area of practice within health care is the use of simple acupressure wrist bands to reduce post-operative nausea and the use of this acupressure point to reduce early morning sickness in pregnancy.

Shiatsu

In common with Chinese acupuncture and acupressure the Japanese therapy of shiatsu attempts to balance energy flow (qi). Shiatsu uses a diagnostic examination of the back or abdomen as guidance for the practitioner.

Also in common with acupressure, pressure is used, usually via the fingers although this could be via the hands, elbows, knees or feet on particular points. The client usually lies down on a padded mattress. This enables 90° pressure to be exerted using gravity rather than additional force.

As direct pressure is applied the contraindications for massage also apply to shiatsu so it should not be used over fractures, burns, wounds, broken skin, varicose veins, or operation sites. Shiatsu should always be delivered by a qualified practitioner who can advise of the contraindications.

Case study: Shiatsu
by Anthony Penman

Philip had his appointment to see me made by his wife. He appeared for our first session looking a little tense and uncertain. Philip is aged 53. He has been a university lecturer most of his working life and is now head of department. His contact time with students had decreased and his role was increasingly administrative. Philip is married with three children, the youngest aged 17 and still living at home.

Philip's main concern was a long-term tendency to neck and shoulder tension, particularly evident after a long session in front of the computer. He also had a more recent problem with his right shoulder, which for the last five weeks had been quite stiff and achy, especially in the mornings. He could not link his shoulder problem with any physical event or trauma. He suffered from occasional headaches and from summer hayfever, for which he used an inhaler. He had a history of intermittent lower back problems. He described his back as having 'gone into spasm and seized up' on four or five occasions over a period of 10 years. He never sought medical advice, and each time the problem improved within a day or two. Philip did very little exercise. His wife was a good cook and they tried to eat 'sensibly'. Philip volunteered that he felt he had not been dealing with stress so well of late, and that this had affected his attitude towards work, and caused strains at home.

Session one
Philip had had an aromatherapy massage on holiday, but otherwise had not had body work before. He exhibited a lot of held tension at a deep level. His body was stiff and board-like. His right shoulder was far more locked than his description led me to expect; movement was severely restricted.

Energetically, I worked particularly on his gall bladder, which was very congested (jitsu) and spleen, which was depleted (kyo). A congested gall bladder (jitsu) is often associated with physical stiffness and joint problems.

I went very gently and conservatively with all the stretches. I did not want to give too challenging a treatment when there was so much physical tension and resistance. Gauging this is a matter of judgement and experience. It is important to build trust and I did not want to produce a big reaction to the first session.

At the end Philip was slightly hesitant about booking a session a week hence. I gave him the option to go away and think about it. I explained that he would probably need at least three or four sessions to release his shoulder. He decided to book another session for the following week.

Session two
Philip was more at ease. He reported an improvement in his range of shoulder movement, although there was still restriction and pain taking the arm backwards, as when putting on a shirt or coat. He had slept better the first two nights following his first session, and could sleep on his right side. He had had a fairly light week on the computer, and his neck tension was not too bad.

The gall bladder ki was 'softer' and gall bladder points on the foot less painful when I worked. We discussed again the number and frequency of sessions. I suggested having weekly sessions for four weeks and then to review, possibly moving to two or three-week intervals. I also recommended drinking 1.5–2 litres of water a day for a month, and cutting back on coffee.

Session three
Gardening had upset his shoulder and it had been painful for two days. Philip and his wife had been for a three-mile walk the previous Sunday. He had felt more relaxed at college during the last week, but said his workload had also been lighter. The shoulder was still quite restricted when taking the arm back.

I did soft tissue and energy work around the shoulder-blade and deltoid muscle in both sitting and side-lying positions. Philip relaxed better during this session, although he held his legs rigidly when I performed hip rotations and stretches. He was nearly asleep at the end of the session and I covered him with a blanket for a few minutes.

Session four
Philip was very much lighter in mood and easier with me. He said he was walking differently and was paying more attention to how he sat at the computer. He had had a twinge in his lower back during the previous week, but had been doing some daily stretches, which I had recommended. He felt the stretches had helped to release some tightness in the lower back. His shoulder was 'much improved'. It was less achy, but movement was still restricted. He was still holding his legs tightly during the session. We talked about this, and Philip was able to let me 'have the weight' when I lifted his legs while he was lying on his back. He was still inclined to tighten again at times during the treatment. We discussed further treatment and settled on a three-week interval before the next session.

Session five
Phillip said he had looked forward to the session, but felt that the three-week gap was a bit too long and booked his next session for two weeks later.

Follow up
Philip continues to come for shiatsu when he feels he is 'tightening up' – about once a month on average. He has used some ibuprofen gel on his right shoulder and has now regained full range of movement. He continues with his stretching routine most days, and says he feels physically more supple. He has had no more 'episodes' with his back, and his headaches have not returned.

He feels his concentration has improved and he is more easily able to relax in the evenings at home. He and his wife now go on some quite ambitious walks. Philip says he does not know if it is the shiatsu, but he feels that he is coping better with unforeseen events at work and he is able to take a more flexible approach with colleagues.

(Reproduced with kind permission from www.webhealth.co.uk.
Accessed 14 December 2005)

Kinesiology

According to kinesiology theory, muscle dysfunction reflects imbalance within the body. Based on a theory of energy meridians similar to acupuncture it is seen that where there is an imbalance this will correspond to muscle weakness.

During a consultation, different large muscles are selected and pressed by the practitioner while the client tries to maintain certain positions. If the muscle is 'weak' there will be no resistance; if it is 'strong' it will be easy to keep in position.

Foods, chemicals, herbal and homeopathic remedies can also be tested by holding them against the body, or by having them in the mind during testing. The substance or thought is believed to exert an influence on the body 'circuits', influencing muscle function.

Kinesiology is used particularly in the assessment and treatment of long-standing conditions.

Case study: Kinesiology
By Anne-Lise Miller

Lisa came to see me with severe knee pain. She had a hospital appointment six weeks later to have both her knees cut open and scraped. At the age of 63 she runs a wildlife rescue centre and has a very physically demanding daily schedule of feeding and cleaning the animals in her care. Her knees were so painful she was desperate to find a way of managing the pain so she could carry on looking after her animals.

During her first appointment she expressed her determination to follow all of my suggestions and to trust the process fully. For that reason I was able to go straight into the therapy without wasting time building her trust.

The first three sessions were spaced one week apart and I concentrated on strengthening the muscles supporting the knees (sartorius, quadriceps, gracilis, bicep femoris, etc.). The main overall emerging picture was that with her stress levels being high her adrenals were exhausted. She needed nutritional support so I also recommended she ate small and often and cut out sugar and caffeine.

On her fourth visit she announced that she had cancelled her hospital appointment because her pain and general well-being were so much better. However, she still felt some pain at certain times of the day and I decided to concentrate more specifically on the inflammation causing the pain. I tested her food sensitivities and found her to be sensitive to dairy and wheat. I also found that she responded positively to antibiotic herbs. She phoned me three days later and said that she was climbing the walls with the cravings and that her knees felt a lot worse. I encouraged her to carry on and a week latter she phoned again to tell me that she was practically pain free. Since then Lisa has been coming for regular maintenance treatments and is feeling stronger and fitter than she has done for years.

(Reproduced with kind permission from www.webhealth.co.uk.
Accessed 14 December 2005)

Iridology

Developed in the 19th century in Hungary, iridology is a diagnostic method using magnification and examination of the iris in order to diagnose health problems.

It is believed that the iris relates to specific areas of the body and, in a similar way in which reflexology maps the body against hands and feet, the iridologist maps the six segmented rings of the iris to parts of the body. The thousands of nerve endings in the iris are thought to relay nerve messages from the brain and this is used to identify problems in different parts of the body. The patterns and changes within the iris are thought to reflect the modified nerve messages returning from the brain. Changes may be seen as markings on the iris that differ from those markings that are inherited.

In particular, iridology particularly focuses on the organs of elimination such as the liver, skin, lungs, lymphatic system, kidneys and bladder. Iridology does not necessarily claim to diagnose specific problems but rather to identify weaknesses. For example, problems with elimination or absorption of nutrients may be detected in the iris. Examination of the eye includes the pupil and the changes that may occur here. Iridologists may use pupil size to determine faulty nerve impulses from the spinal cord.

Training, education and regulation

Training is based in a number of colleges. The Guild of Naturopathic Iridologists International advises on training and on accredited members. Guild members also work in accordance with a professional code of ethics and hold professional indemnity insurance.

Uses within health care

In some European universities iridology is taught to medical students and in the USA there is at least one professorship in iridology. It is viewed within these organizations that iridology will become an integrated diagnostic tool. However, there is much debate within the medical profession about the validity of iridology.

Case study: Iridology
by Harriet Di Luzio

This case study concerns a happily married young lady, 34 years of age, with a bubbly infectious personality who is extremely good with people and who loves to chat. You could not fail to like her as she always has a smile on her face.

She has a responsible job with an international airline. She thoroughly enjoys her job, but the downside was shift work which included late nights, sometimes followed by very early morning starts. She usually worked a six days on and three days off rota. She is a non-smoker and a very occasional social drinker, only at birthdays, Christmas and family occasions.

Her presenting symptoms were recorded by the iris analysis done at the time, which showed the following:

■   Severe headaches.
■   Stress rings.
■   Immune system depletion.
■   Elimination problems from lymphatic system and digestive system.
■   Endocrine weakness/irregular periods.
■   Exhaustion.
■   Depleted nervous system.
■   Indications of insufficient fluid intake.

This young lady desperately wanted a baby. She had had two miscarriages and one pregnancy that had resulted in the birth of a child during the fifth month of pregnancy but baby died shortly after. Eighteen months later she had an ectopic pregnancy, which resulted in surgery at 10 weeks, whereupon her right fallopian tube was removed. She kept her right ovary. Her doctor had introduced folic acid into her regime.

I spoke to her gently about examining her left then right iris telling her that I would talk her through what I found. I also asked her if she was open to suggestions, to which she eagerly agreed, such was her desire to be a mother.

The really interesting aspect of iridology is that, by examining each iris, you get first hand information concerning the level of toxins in the body, where they are and what bodily system they are having an effect on. Here I found there was poor elimination from the bowels and a poor blood circulatory system leading to an inefficient immune and lymphatic system.

My immediate reaction was to deal with elimination from the bowels. Unless this system began working this young lady would find things difficult. She had the added problem of always putting off a motion: If she felt the urge to open her bowels at the workplace she said it was difficult to leave her station as it needed a supervisor to take over from her. This, it appeared, was standard practice. In addition she also neglected to have any form of liquid refreshment for the same reason.

We discussed her options and decided that unless the stagnation in the bowel was eliminated, exhaustion would continue to be a problem. She readily agreed to be part of her own treatment. The next day she bought a pure bristle body brush and began to enhance the circulation of the blood, with dry skin brushing. Following this with hot then cold showers she immediately began to have a spring in her step and actually began to look forward to the start of her day wherever that was in her work shift pattern. She also began to take herbs for the bowels. The herbs in this formula included buckthorn, cascara, cayenne, clover, coughgrass, dandelion, ginger, liquorice, and lobelia. I have not included details of the amounts of herbs, as this differs between patients and practitioners. An immediate effect was felt from this formula and after a week the severe headaches she had experienced began to subside. The initial response to treatment was encouraging as toxins began to be eliminated.

Constitutional strengths and weaknesses can be seen in the iris. This particular lady was prone to allergies, swollen glands, skin eruptions, eye irritations, calcium deficiency and weak glands, namely the thyroid and adrenals as well as a sensitive nervous system. Therefore she tended to be somewhat anxious at times. Relaxation appeared to be something that she did not do much of, complaining of not having enough time for anything except work.

Weekly sessions of reflexology began to take place. The first session was getting to know the feet, as some people find it very odd having their feet touched by another person. It took a little while for the lady to allow herself to relax, and when she did relax it was quite noticeable. All areas of the feet were tense, perhaps in anticipation. I told her to drink plenty of water until I saw her the next week, as this would prove beneficial.

The following session was scheduled for a week later with her more tender points being the thoracic and transverse colon both on the right medial side. At the end of the treatment she looked pale and asked for a moment to herself. When she had composed herself she mentioned that her first session the previous week had caused her a headache. However, later, when she had been seeing me for about eight weeks, she had only had one headache, whereas normally she was getting three a week. One could consider that the herbs were working on one level and the reflexology on another but both were having a therapeutic result.

Her last period had been in March and her next period was now 26 days late. She had done a pregnancy test, which proved negative. She wanted to know when was the best time to start trying for a baby. Again I spoke to her about proper dietary habits; and not having the odd snack here and there instead of a meal. She readily agreed that she was still not eating properly and had failed to get into any sort of routine when it came to eating. This I felt was an area that caused her great anxiety because of her constant worry about when or where she would be, and in what situation she should find herself, when she may need the toilet. I continued to encourage her to eat better and praised her when she did.

At her next reflexology appointment in June she had still had no period. She had been free of pain until the day before her appointment, at which time the pain had come and just gone again.

Herbs for the cleansing of the reproductive system were given. These included squaw vine, raspberry leaves, cayenne, golden seal and cramp bark. Squaw vine was bought to us via the North American Indians and is said to be one of the best remedies for preparing the uterus for child bearing along with raspberry leaves whose actions include strengthening and toning the tissues of the womb. Cayenne, which is one of the most useful systemic stimulants, strengthens the heart and arteries, as well as being a powerful circulatory herb thereby regulating the blood flow. Golden seal's action is that of a tonic, astringent, and muscular stimulant and, as it can stimulate the involuntary muscles of the uterus, it is to be avoided in pregnancy. Cramp bark is both an anti-spasmodic and a sedative. It relieves painful cramps associated with the menstrual cycle, a symptom that the patient had been experiencing in the past. Once again no specifics about the dosage are given here as doses differ between patients and practitioners.

Reflexology treatments continued and one in particular was of great interest to her. Working on her left foot at the uterus point she reported feeling warmth along what she called her bikini line and she felt this held some significance. I worked her tender areas on the right foot, including the lymphatic drainage point, the breast and diaphragm.

Reflexology now became fortnightly as her work schedule changed. The next session two weeks later found her coming in with heavy swollen glands. My thoughts were that we should still be having weekly sessions as the swollen glands were showing me how important it was to keep regular sessions going in a person with erratic working hours and dietary intake. However her bowel motions had changed to being very moist so there was a little improvement which showed her that things can change when you begin to eat properly. She continued to be stressed due to overwork and working shifts and she was thinking of taking a holiday in two months time. This was a breakthrough as it was the first time she had put herself first.

She was beginning to realize that if she did not finally learn to relax her body would always be in a state of anxiety, which could lead to more severe problems in the future. It felt to me that a breakthrough had occurred and the uphill battle was turning itself around. I admire people who make the decision to change their lifestyle patterns, especially where health is an issue, but I also know that when the time is right for that individual they will be ready. We are all individuals with emotions and feelings that have to be worked through first in our own minds before we find the path we need to follow, to make our new decision a success.

Having made that decision helped to relax this lady and when she came for her next reflexology session she happily announced that she had now had a period, three months after the last, which had a good flow and lasted a week. Two days previously she said it was a hot muggy day and she had felt head pains originating at the back of her head, but she felt good at the end of this reflexology session.

She announced that the reflexology sessions would become fewer due to work commitments, although she had made a conscious decision to continue coming to collect the herbs for the reproductive system, bowels and circulation. This continued until November when she arrived feeling extremely tired, with both feet aching. The only tender areas on her feet were on the left, those connected to the kidney, bladder and lower back. We again discussed fluid intake and the importance of the required amount of daily fluids, especially water. But this is not what was on her mind. She wanted to talk about the eptopic pregnancy she had had a few years previously. She was worried that the herbs she is taking would interfere with her menstrual cycle. She felt her biological clock was rapidly ticking away.

With regard to the herbs interfering with her cycle, I had spoken to her about this when we first met, when I had suggested putting a time limit on taking them. We had agreed when she first came to me that we would review her progress at the end of the year. We now therefore reviewed the situation and what had been achieved. In March she had had a period, with the next in June. Her period in August was 30 days late, in September 9 days late, in November 18 days late, and in December it was 10 days late. She was now free of the pain previously experienced during her periods.

Her bowel motions had improved, with the help of the bowel herbs, as had the appearance and texture of her skin. Reflexology had alerted her to the need to relax the mind, body and spirit if she wishes to keep her body in balance.

We had discussed the length of time we would spend enhancing the endocrine system and the elimination process and were now ready to stop all herbs. I sensed she was uncertain about this but I explained that there are herbs that are contra-indicated in pregnancy and we should consider this now.

As she left she promised to let me know how things went and I was pleased to receive a call three months later telling me she was pregnant. Once again we began meeting for her to have reflexology as a relaxant as well as keeping the nerve and blood supply enhanced. She had a baby girl in December that year.

Reference

Rankin Box D (2001) *The Nurses Handbook of Complementary Therapies.* London: Bailliere Tindall

Further reading and sources of information

Iridology
The Guild of Naturopathic Iridologists International. Website: www.gni-international.org

Kinesiology
Kinesiology Federation, PO Box 28909, Dalkeith EH22 2YQ

Tel: 0870 011 3545

www.kinesiologyfederation.org

Schiatsu
www.webhealth.co.uk

Chapter 5

Therapies in focus:
Aromatherapy, Bach flower remedies, reflexology, massage therapy, Alexander technique and Bowen therapy

Aromatherapy

What is it?

Aromatherapy is the controlled use of the extracted essential oils from plants in order to maintain and/or improve the health of mind, body and spirit.

For centuries a wide range of cultures have used the healing properties of essential oils. The Egyptians use oils of myrrh, clove and others to embalm bodies. The oils were also used to make perfumes and in religious ceremonies. In ancient China extracts of plants were used for their medicinal purposes and the traditional form of Indian medicine, ayurveda, also uses plant extracts. Biblical references to essential oils illustrate the history of essential oils within religion.

It was however during the 1920s when chemist Gattefosse used lavender oil to ease the pain of a chemical burn that interest in the medicinal properties of oils began to increase. The term aromatherapy was introduced to Britain from Europe in the 1950s by Marguerite Maury and since this time its use has grown rapidly.

The general public have become accustomed to essential oils in pharmaceutical products, and hair care and home cleaning products. Essential oils are available in supermarkets and chemists across the UK.

An essential oil is an aromatic, non-greasy plant extract composed only of the volatile molecules from the plant concerned. The essential oil may be extracted from the flowers, leaves, bark or resin. Methods of extraction vary as does the quality of the oil. Essential oils are diluted for use with a 'carrier' which may be an oil, a lotion or alcohol. The choice of carrier will depend on the method of application.

The most common methods of application are:

- Massage with a carrier oil/lotion.
- Compress.

Table 5.1: Main uses of commonly used essential oils			
Essential oil	Main uses	Warnings	Application
Lavender	Soothing and relaxing, refreshing, burns, boils, nervous tension, insomnia rheumatism	None	Massage, inhalation, baths, compress
Tea tree	Antiseptic, anti-viral, cold sores, verrucae, athletes foot, colds and flu, head lice	None	Massage
Geranium	Balancing, depression, anxiety, dry eczema, skin care, hormonal balance	None	Massage, baths
Neroli	Nervous tension, insomnia	None	Massage, baths
Chamomile	Calming, menopause, arthritis and rheumatism, anxiety, inflamed skin	None	Massage, compress
Rosemary	Diuretic, headache, arthritis, colds and flu, mental stimulation	Epilepsy, pregnancy	Massage, inhalation, baths
Sandalwood	Soothing/skin care, bronchitis, cough, catarrh, dry eczema	None	Massage, inhalation, baths
Peppermint	Cooling, digestion, headaches, nausea, travel sickness	Skin sensitivity	Inhalation, compress/ massage after skin test
Ylang-ylang	Psychological, panic, irrationality, shyness aphrodisiac	None	Massage, baths

- Inhalation/vaporization.
- Bath.

It is suggested that the essential oils affect the individual on both a physical and psychological level. The chemical components of the essential oils are absorbed by the body through the skin when applied in a carrier. This has been compared to the action of products like hormone replacement patches. The essential oils may also be absorbed via inhalation whereby the chemical components are absorbed via the lungs. The olfactory nerves also carry messages from the receptors in the nose to the hypothalamus and the limbic system controlling emotional aspects of behaviour. Psychologically it has been suggested that aroma plays an important role in memory and it is also suggested that the chemical components of the essential oils are known to cause a relaxation response. A well-known example of this is the use of lavender oil to induce sleep. An aromatherapist will treat a client taking into account physical and psychological symptoms holistically and choose oils to benefit the client.

Table 5.1 identifies commonly used oils with some of their main properties and contraindications. It is important to bear in mind though that all essential oils can cause skin sensitivity in some individuals so all essential oils must be diluted before use on the skin.

Safety and contraindications

Most essential oils are generally safe if used in a dilution of under 4%. However, oils should be used with caution and under the advice of a qualified aromatherapist in pregnant women and in those with epilepsy, high blood pressure or diabetes.

Essential oils should never be taken internally. Some essential oils can be irritants. In general, essential oils should never be used undiluted on the skin, although there is evidence to demonstrate the safe use of undiluted lavender oil for burns. However, even when diluted some individuals may be sensitive to some oils.

It is important to recognize the safety aspects of using essential oils. Many patients may use them within their own homes but within the health care environment essential oils should always be used under the guidance of a qualified aromatherapist.

Training, education and regulation

Training as an aromatherapist is available in a number of universities, colleges and private sector organizations. However, there is currently no specific requirement by law to complete a specific course or register with a specific organization. The Aromatherapy Consortium provides an umbrella organization with the aim of developing a single register for voluntary registration and common standards for training.

Uses within health care

A number of studies have identified the use of aromatherapy with specific client groups. These studies include the use of lavender essential oil with foot massage in cardiac patients in intensive care (Woolfson and Hewitt, 1994). This study suggested that the use of essential oils with massage led to a lowering of blood pressure, heart rate and respiratory rate. Within the area of palliative care aromatherapy is a popular therapy with a number of studies supporting its use in a range of situations including symptom control in cancer patients (Kohn, 2000).

Within the field of mental health the studies are more limited but a number highlight the potential of aromatherapy to aid relaxation, enhance mood and reduce anxiety in specific clients (Borotoft, 1996; Jelinek and Novakora, 2001; Field et al, 1993; Edge, 2003). Certain essential oils have been associated with the relief of some symptoms of dementia (Burns et al, 2002). Aromatherapy has been used extensively by nurses caring for individuals with profound and multiple learning disabilities. Studies have identified the therapeutic effects of essential oils and massage. Midwifery has used aromatherapy in a range of areas and studies highlight the uses of essential oils pre- and post-natally.

Case study: Aromatherapy
by Nicky Genders

Mary is a 51-year-old who came for an aromatherapy treatment after her GP had suggested massage as a form of relaxation. While taking a detailed medical history and asking about her physical state, Mary identified that she felt her anxiety stemmed from her role as a carer for her disabled mother. Her main symptoms included difficulty in sleeping, general tension-type headaches and very dry skin. Mary was also menopausal and this was causing a range of symptoms including mood swings and feelings of 'panic'. Due to a previous medical condition Mary was not able to use hormone replacement therapy. Mary suggested her diet was fairly healthy and she regularly took vitamin and mineral supplements.

Using the detailed history and considering Mary's current symptoms I mixed a blend of the following essential oils to support both her physical and psychological symptoms.

1. *Lavender*: Useful for insomnia, tension headaches, irritability, mood swings, worry and panic attacks.
2. *Geranium*: Useful for hormonal imbalance, dry skin, mood swings.
3. *Chamomile Roman*: Useful for gentle soothing of a restless mind.

Mary liked the aroma so this blend was diluted into sweet almond oil to use for massage. In addition to the massage oil Mary also took the blend home in a base for use in the bath and a small amount of the blend for inhalation, particularly useful for the feelings of panic.

Mary had a fortnightly back massage for around four months and currently has a monthly back massage. She reported using the bath base twice weekly and the blend for inhalation whenever she felt a 'bit panicky'. During this time she has reported that she slept better, particularly after using the blend in the bath. She also reported that she found it easier to cope with her menopausal symptoms, and the mood swings seemed to have evened out. She had no feelings of panic after the first month of treatment. In addition her headaches had all but disappeared. Mary's skin had improved in texture and much of the dryness had gone.

It is clear, in Mary's case, that the combination of massage and essential oils reduced her psychological problems.

Bach flower remedies

In addition to aromatherapy other complementary therapies exist which use extracted essences of plant materials. Two of the best known are Australian bush essences and, more commonly used in the UK, Bach flower essences.

Dr Edward Bach, using his knowledge of homeopathy, developed a series of remedies using extracted flower essences in the 1930s with the philosophy that the remedies work by stimulating the body's own healing response. Using a link between a healthy mind and a healthy body Dr Bach devised a system of emotional groups in order to classify people. These seven emotional groups included fear, uncertainty, and oversensitivity. Within each of these categories a further 38 negative feelings were identified with a corresponding remedy for each. The remedies are generally diluted in water and taken as needed. Up to seven different remedies can be taken at one time. The most common remedy combination is a pre-mixed combination called Rescue Remedy. This mixture of rock rose, *impatiens*, clematis, star of Bethlehem and cherry plum is used by many to deal with pre-exam or test nerves, general shock and to provide focus for a current difficult task. *Table 5.2* lists all 38 remedies and their uses.

Table 5.2: Bach remedies and their uses

Category	Negative feeling	Bach flower remedy
Fear	Terror	Rock rose
	Fear of unknown	Mimulus
	Fear of mind giving way	Cherry plum
	Fears/worries of unknown origin	Aspen
	Fear/over-concern for others	Red chestnut
Loneliness	Pride/aloofness	Water violet
	Impatience	*Impatiens*
	Self-centredness/self-concern	Heather
Insufficient interest in present circumstances	Dreaminess/lack of interest in present	Clematis
	Lives in the past	Honeysuckle
	Resignation/apathy	Wild rose
	Lack of energy	Olive
	Unwanted thoughts/mental arguments	White chestnut
	Deep gloom with no apparent origin	Mustard
	Failure to learn from past mistakes	Chestnut bud
Despondency or despair	Lack of confidence	Larch
	Self-reproach/guilt	Pine
	Overwhelmed by responsibility	Elm
	Extreme mental anguish	Sweet chestnut
	After-effects of shock	Star of Bethlehem
	Resentment	Willow
	Exhausted but struggles on	Oak
	Self-hatred/sense of uncleanliness	Crab apple
Uncertainty	Seeks advice and confirmation from others	*Cerato*
	Indecision	*Scleranthus*
	Discouragement/despondency	Gentian
	Hopelessness and despair	Gorse
	'Monday morning' feeling	Hornbeam
	Uncertainty about life path	Wild oat

Oversensitivity to influences and ideas	Mental torment but putting on a brave face	Agrimony
	Subservient and weak willed	Centaury
	Protection from change and outside influences	Walnut
	Jealousy/hatred/envy	Holly
Over-concern for the welfare of others	Selfish possessiveness	Chicory
	Over-enthusiasm	Vervain
	Domineering/inflexible	Vine
	Intolerance	Beech
	Self-repression/self-denial	Rock water

Case study: Bach flower remedy
by Beth Tyers

A baby boy was delivered by Ventouse intervention after a long and traumatic labour. His mother had some assistance with homeopathy, administered by her husband. Sleep had been impossible for all of the baby's 15 or 16 days of life. He had a large haematoma to the back and one side of his head. Feeding was difficult, stressful for both mother and baby, as the baby could not relax enough to latch on successfully.

Homeopathic remedies were given and successfully reduced the haematoma but the baby still could not rest and was agitated, twitching, stretching and straining and spending very little time still. He seemed to respond normally to his father's and mother's voices, and all of his reflexes were assessed as normal. He became distressed if his head was touched. He passed normal quantities of urine and stools, but was not gaining weight at the rate expected.

Remedies given in sequence were *Arnica, Nat. sulph, Stramonium, Helleborus, Cicuta, Chamomilla,* and *Colocynth,* without noticeable effect on his general state.

His mother rang in the third week after birth, in tears of desperation, at about 10.30 p.m. one evening. The baby had been screaming uncontrollably, unable to feed or sleep. There was no possibility of getting any remedies to her quickly (other than those she had in her first aid and birth kits, and those already tried). My advice at this point was for the mother and baby to get into a warm bath with a large squirt of Rescue Remedy in the water, and to massage Rescue Remedy into baby's hands and feet. I asked her to call me the next day, when I would have more time to discuss the next step.

She did phone next morning, in tears again, this time with relief, saying that they had all slept through the night for the first time since the birth. The effect had been immediate – the baby had relaxed considerably in the bath, fed well and then slept. He had fed well again that morning and was sleeping again. She asked me what she should do next. My advice was to repeat the massage twice daily into the hands and feet and repeat the shared Rescue Remedy bath each evening.

Clearly the Rescue Remedy had broken the vicious cycle of tension that was contributing to the baby's condition. As mother was becoming more and more desperate each day, she, too, needing calming. I feel, however, that the flower essence affected the baby's energy on a very deep level indeed, relieving the immense shock of the traumatic delivery and enabling rest, digestion, and the proper assimilation of later homeopathic remedies, all of which worked effectively, and continue to do so. He is now a happy, healthy 3-year-old.

(Reproduced with kind permission from www.webhealth.co.uk.
Accessed 14 December 2005)

Reflexology

What is it

First practised by the Chinese, Indians and Egyptians the ancient art of reflexology is described as a gentle holistic balancing treatment that will help to increase energy levels, ease aches and pains, reduce levels of stress, relax the body and calm the mind

Reflexology is based on the view that the body is made up of 10 energy zones. It is suggested that within the feet, hands and ears there are reflex points corresponding to all organs, glands and parts of the body, i.e. the feet are mirrors reflecting the condition of the body. Due to injury, stress, or illness the body can end up in a state of imbalance and vital energy pathways can be blocked which can prevent the body from functioning properly.

This division of the body into energy zones or meridians is similar to the mapping used within acupuncture and acupressure. The reflexologist works with the understanding that when a meridian point is blocked then the energy flow becomes abnormal and congestion may occur at that point. The view is that reflexology can be used to remove these blockages and correct the balance.

Reflex points have been mapped on both the hands and feet and these correspond to areas and organs of the body (see *Figure 5.1*).

By using specific finger and thumb pressure reflexology stimulates and frees energy by helping to release blockages within the body, enabling the body to heal itself. When working, the reflexologist may find areas at the reflex points that feel grainy or tense. Applying pressure to the areas will then 'unblock' energy and assist the body's own healing mechanism.

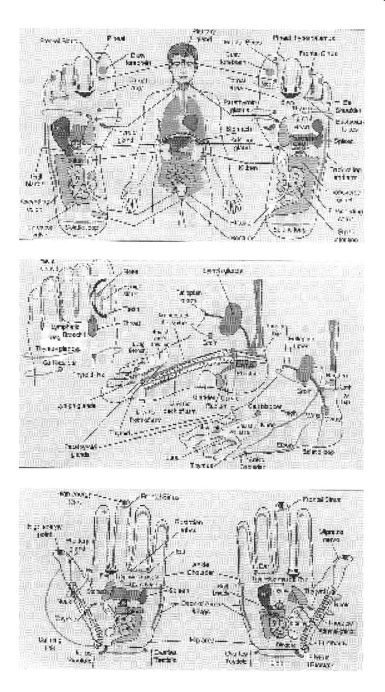

Figure 5.1: Top: reflex areas of the feet, with the body parts to which they correspond.. Middle: Reflex areas of the feet showing their symmetry. Bottom: Reflex areas of the hand.

It is suggested that almost everyone can benefit from reflexology as it treats the entire body rather than just the symptoms of disease and can be used to bring relief to a wide range of acute as well as chronic problems including:

- Joint and muscle pain.
- Gastrointestinal problems.
- Skin problems.
- Menstrual problems.

Training, education and regulation

A number of training courses exist within higher and further education to train as a reflexologist. However, it is not a requirement by law to undertake any of these courses. There are a number of associations working together under the umbrella organization, the Reflexology Forum, which accredit courses and keep registers of members.

Uses in health care

There has been a rising popularity among patients for reflexology treatments and a growing evidence base supporting its use for a variety of conditions, including:

- Pre-menstrual syndrome (Peters et al, 2002).
- Multiple sclerosis (Joyce and Richardson, 1997).
- Palliative care (Wright et al, 2002).
- Midwifery practice (Tiran, 1996).

Reflexology is being offered in some pain clinics and hospices as part of care packages. However, health professionals do need to be aware that there are contraindications for reflexology treatment including diabetes, circulatory problems and epilepsy. A trained reflexologist will be able to advise on appropriate treatment.

Case study: Reflexology
by Maggie Brooks

Eleanor agreed to act as a case study. She felt she was fine with no real problems; she could unwind as necessary and slept well. Her husband had given her a gift voucher and suggested that she try reflexology as he felt she would benefit, having experienced it himself. Indeed, his chronic sinusitis had eased after one session and was no longer a problem after another two sessions.

Eleanor, aged 47, is a staff nurse in an intensive care unit which, although stressful at times, she enjoys. She also works three evenings a week at a private hospital for extra money. This she found less stressful but her workload is considerable. Her husband works part-time due to some health problems which had meant retraining. He hopes to return to full-time work by the end of the year. It has been a difficult few years and this had taken its toll, but Eleanor feels she is coping and that the bad days are truly over. Her son, James (age 20) is studying medicine and lives in a flat while daughter Jan (age 18) is living at home and is a hairdresser. Eleanor's family live in the south of Scotland and both her parents are well.

Primary complaint
In the first instance, Eleanor felt she did not have any complaints, certainly not that anything could be done about. The first consultation in reflexology includes detailed questioning, which is necessary if we are to embark on truly holistic care of a client. Eleanor felt her only problem was constant back pain that she did not feel anything could be done about. She had real problems with her right hip but had seen no point in getting any kind of treatment as nothing would work.

It later came out that she also suffered from severe irritable bowel syndrome (IBS). She admitted her diet was not good and she had put on 2 stone over the last couple of years. The problem was carry-out fish suppers and ice cream on her late shifts. She smoked about 20–25 cigarettes a day. There was no time for any social life, and she preferred to go to bed early.

At her consultation, I recorded no past medical history apart from some reconstructive surgery to her nose 15 years ago. Eleanor is still menstruating normally.

Goals of treatment
I felt I had to 'go extremely canny' with Eleanor. Too many suggestions all at once would frighten her away. I hoped that we could improve her back, and at the same time her IBS. As she had not had any other treatment, I was also very interested to see what reflexology could do for back pain when used on its own without massage or osteopathy. She had resisted any suggestions in regard to those treatments. She looked tired but was cheery and ready to be looked after.

First treatment
I always inspect the client's feet on the first appointment. Eleanor's feet were a little callused on the right but otherwise, apart from being pale, were all right. As usual I began by working on her toes (after the warm up). She found this fascinating and was surprised at how the different reflexes elicited different sensations.

The head areas on the right foot were more tender than on the left. The lumbar areas were exquisitely tender on both feet; L5 more on the left, L4 more on the right. The knee area and the hip (even more so) on the right side were also tender. I could see that she had a pelvic tilt when she walked and a lesion at L5. Indeed, the whole spine was tender on both feet. C7/T1 was exquisitely tender on the left; T8–T10 very tender on the right. Her feet were very stiff and unyielding. The pituitary and pineal were more tender on the left; thyroid was more sensitive on the right. The adrenal glands were exquisitely tender. The uterus was more tender on the right and the ovary more tender on the left. The lung areas felt slightly congested, more so on the right, and the liver reflex was tender. The whole bowel area was tender; the ileum on the left was very tender and the colon on the right with the ileo-caecal valve exquisitely tender. The dorsal areas – right elbow, left shoulder – were also very tender. She then told me she often felt her shoulders were tired, tight and sore.

We discussed all this and I showed her the reflexology chart, which she found very interesting. She talked about how busy she was with no time for herself. Her job in intensive care was very hectic. She felt in control and that she rarely got involved with or affected by patients. She felt she could relax easily, and in particular had no problem sleeping. She was however looking forward to a week's holiday.

Eleanor enjoyed her first treatment and was eager for the second. She drank a glass of water after treatment and I suggested she start a new habit. She thought this was strange but agreed to try it. We agreed to meet again in one week's time to allow her body to adjust to what we had done. I warned her that she might show signs and symptoms of toxicity, such as headache and/or fatigue and just to treat it with rest and drinking water.

Second treatment - one week later
Eleanor returned saying she had been looking forward to her next treatment. She had felt well, been sleeping better and was impressed. What had amazed Eleanor most was that she felt that she was less stiff, although she would have expected to be more so, as she was on holiday and had been stripping paper off the bathroom walls.

We discussed diet. Eleanor said she did not have time to make a packed lunch or dinner as she felt she already had more than enough to do. Rice Krispies were the one thing that eased her IBS. Eleanor did not want to discuss personal issues and I respected this.

We used the session to relax. The right hip area was still exquisitely tender, but the thoracic area had improved as had the cervical area. The elbow and shoulder areas had also improved. and I was surprised and delighted.

We discussed drinking less caffeine and more water and taking a short walk every day. We agreed to meet in one week's time.

Third treatment - one week later
Eleanor was moving more easily and was feeling better in herself. She admitted that she had not realized how stressed she had got. Her husband had commented that she was looking younger. (Indeed he had told me how pleased he was that she was finally taking some time for herself.)

We continued the session, working the spinal and musculoskeletal areas as before. I increased the mobilizations of her feet as she could now tolerate more. The bowel area had improved quite dramatically from the first visit. She reported that her colic had eased so much she was able to forget about it at times. Eleanor's feet were now more flexible and looked better in regard to texture and colour.

We discussed home treatment but she felt she wouldn't have time and preferred to come to see me. Some clients like to work on hand reflexes to complement what is happening at the treatment. We agreed to meet in two weeks' time.

Fourth treatment - two weeks later
Eleanor continued to feel that she had more energy and her mobility was improving. She felt that the pain in her hip was lessening and her lower back was moving much more easily. She agreed that as her pain decreased, she would be more likely to consider going for a walk.

The nervous and endocrine points were tender as follows: cervical on the right, particularly C6 and C7; T1 on the right, T4 on the left, T8 on the right, T12 on the right; L3, L5 and sacrum on the right; pituitary on the right; thymus on the left; adrenal on the right; and ovary on the right. The lung areas seemed more congested this time and when I mentioned it she said she had found that after the previous treatments, she had been smoking less but her smoking had been on the increase again over the previous three days. However, it had reduced overall. The stomach was more tender than on the previous visit and I felt this was related to the lung congestion. The bowel areas were again very tender, particularly on the left over the hepatic flexure and transverse colon.

We included some breathing techniques, which she enjoyed. The session was mainly relaxation. Eleanor obviously enjoyed just being herself and not 'on call' for this hour. She volunteered that she planned on cutting down on smoking and told me that her overall diet had improved slightly. We agreed to meet again in three weeks time.

Fifth treatment - three weeks later
Eleanor felt there was a definite improvement in her hip and lower back, so much so that she was enjoying going for a short walk each day. This was a dramatic change, particularly as Eleanor did feel constantly under time constraints. She had cut down

on smoking, which she was proud of and delighted about. She was feeling tired and was looking forward to being re-energized again.

The right hip and spinal areas were the most tender, more the lumbar and lower thoracics. C7/T1 was still tender (about 4 out of 5) on the right. This junction is a vulnerable area for everyone. Eleanor's feet relaxed more easily than at her previous treatments suggesting an overall improvement in her ability to relax. She reported that her bowel was fine now and that she really had no other problems. We agreed to meet in six weeks.

Sixth treatment - six weeks later
Eleanor was well. The pelvic tilt I spotted at the first visit was still apparent, but not as much. She remained delighted with her improved musculoskeletal system. She had also surprised herself with her continued progress and now looked forward to another session. We worked as before and I noted the overall improvement in all the points. Hip and lumbar spine were still tender (about 3–4 out of 5). She opened up a little about the hard times she had had and then said she felt she had handled all she needed to handle. I absolutely respect the client's right to privacy, and, in this case, I was aware too, that starting to talk might well open up a lot of issues that would require specialized counselling and, at the same time, might also prevent her from working. As the major breadwinner, this was something that she could choose to do in her own time. I mentioned to her how past events and issues can affect health quite dramatically and she agreed.

We concluded the reflexology treatment with some breathing and lymphatic pump techniques. Eleanor stated how glad she was that she had come for treatment as she had benefited so much. She also had decided to continue with reflexology on a regular basis for as long as she needed it.

Seventh treatment - eight weeks later
Eight weeks had passed since her last treatment, and Eleanor had found that her hip was at last easing a bit to the point where it was not painful all the time. She was smoking less, still drinking more water and had lost 2 kg in weight. She was also feeling more like her 'old self' and she and her husband had gone out several times, once with friends.

The treatment went well. Eleanor was tired and happy to relax as work had been very busy. The adrenal areas were more sensitive than they had been on the last visit. The spinal areas were still tender but now she scored 2 out of 5 and occasionally 3. The hip still scored higher than the rest.

She promised to attend in a couple of months for another treatment. She hoped to be able to tell me that she had lost more weight.

Conclusion

Eleanor had really only come for reflexology to please her husband. She had expected it to be a nice experience and was astounded at the effects. Her back pain along with her hip pain had gone. Her irritable bowel syndrome was no longer a problem. She did not feel as stressed and lacking in energy. Indeed, the increased awareness she had developed in response to her reflexology treatments had let her realize how low she had got. Eleanor continues with a very busy schedule and manages to come for reflexology about once or twice a year. As an osteopath, I was amazed at the effects that reflexology could have on back pain. Originally, I had advised Eleanor to have osteopathy but she had declined.

Massage

What is it?

Touch has its roots in earliest history as a means of healing and comfort. It is mentioned in Greek mythology, and civilizations from ancient Egypt to native Indians all identify touch as a means to heal.

Massage as a therapy has existed for centuries, across many cultures. In the West massage as a therapy was particularly popular in the late 19th and early 20th century. In 1884 a group of British women formed the Society of Trained Masseuses and this group later became the Chartered Society of Physiotherapists (Horrigan cited in Rankin Box, 2001).

Both World Wars saw nurses using therapeutic massage but, as technology increased, the use of massage (and other forms of therapeutic touch) declined. Massage has in recent decades increased in popularity and its use within health care is well documented.

Massage involves the use of soft tissue manipulation for the benefit of the whole person. It is seen to improve circulation, relax muscles and increase lymphatic drainage (Maxwell Hudson, 1996). Massage may be included within an aromatherapy treatment or may focus on particular areas of the body, for example, Indian head massage. There are many forms of massage and most forms used in the West incorporate some elements of Swedish body massage. A range of movements are incorporated within therapeutic massage and these include:

- *Effleurage*: relaxing and stretching the superficial muscles of the body.
- *Petrissage*: kneading and squeezing of superficial and deeper muscles and soft tissue.
- *Friction*: movements that break down the adhesions between tissues and relax muscle fibres.
- *Tapotement*: percussive strokes aimed at increasing blood flow.

Generally one massage treatment will include some or all of these movements. A trained massage therapist will chose appropriate movements dependent upon the client's needs and health condition.

There has been much debate about the contraindications for massage but many of these can be overcome by professionally trained therapists who are able to adapt technique.

Uses within health care

There are many documented studies demonstrating the use of massage within health care. These studies acknowledge the physiological and psychological benefits of massage (Rankin Box, 2001). Within nursing, one key area is that of palliative care, with studies outlining the use of massage for relaxation, enjoyment, relief from constipation, and analgesia (Ferrell-Torry and Glick, 1993; Flemming, 1997; Gray, 2000; Preece, 2002).

A study by Preece (2002) in the UK demonstrated the efficacy of abdominal massage in a small number of patients in a palliative care setting. Patients in this study reported less discomfort and pain from constipation following a period of regular self-administered abdominal massage.

Within midwifery and health visiting a further area for the use of massage is that of baby massage. A growing body of literature highlights the benefits of this form of massage. Many cultures have a long history of baby massage particularly Malaysia, India and Tibet. It is acknowledged within the literature that baby massage can encourage communication between mother/father and baby, can calm a baby's emotions and aid digestion.

Education, training and regulation

Many courses in both higher and further education exist to train in therapeutic massage, some of these are part of other therapies including aromatherapy.

The General Council for Massage Therapy (GCMT) also has lists of accredited courses. Regulation is currently in the form of self-regulation. Registers exist with the GCMT and other bodies.

Case study: Massage therapy
By Nikki Murray

Introduction
Mrs M is 49 years old and runs her own chiropody business. She is happily married and has two grown up children. In her spare time she enjoys walking, gardening and looking after an array of animals from pheasants and dogs to ferrets.

Presenting problem

For the past few months Mrs M has been suffering from stress. Her chiropody business is very busy, she can sometimes treat up to 15 clients a day. Home visits are her most popular request. Her main signs and symptoms of stress have been a feeling of being overwhelmed, of not being able to sleep at night or to switch off when finished for the day, of being 'crabby' with her family, and she has noticed a loss in her appetite. Her menopausal problems have also been a contributing problem, i.e. headaches and hot flushes.

Consultation

During consultation it was established that Mrs M also suffers from back, neck and shoulder pain from bending over to treat her clients. Also if she over-uses her wrists her (mild) arthritis in her hands and fingers flares up, and the muscles in her forearms are also affected. She has an allergic reaction to aspirin and she is not taking any medication.

Treatment plan

The goals of treatment were to:

- Ease any muscle spasm in the areas causing her pain, i.e. back, neck, shoulders and arms.
- Enable Mrs M to relax.
- Allow Mrs M take some time out for herself.
- Reduce the number of headaches she had been getting.
- Allow her to get a good night's sleep.
- Encourage mobility in hands and fingers.

First visit

We agreed that the primary complaint this time was her aching back and neck. I recommended a back, neck and shoulder massage for the first treatment, which is relaxing as well as easing the muscles that were in spasm.

After the first treatment Mrs M remarked how she felt a load had been lifted off her shoulders and she found her range of movement in her neck had improved and her neck felt much easier.
I advised Mrs M to get a regular massage to really benefit. For her to get some relaxation time for herself would be an additional bonus to the reduction of muscle spasm in her back, neck and shoulders. Feeling more aware and relaxed would have knock-on effects.

Other relaxation techniques were advised, e.g. listening to relaxation tapes, and breathing exercises. Also discussed was the importance of her posture when working and warming up her wrists and fingers before starting work. I suggested exercises to improve general circulation and stretches between clients. I also advised Mrs M to drink at least a litre of water a day when she is busy.

Second visit: one week later

Mrs M had a busy week with her regular clients, so she reported that her back, neck and shoulders had begun to ache again. However, she had felt better, slept better, felt more refreshed but was becoming more agitated again.

Once again her back, neck and shoulders were massaged. There were areas of tight muscles mainly on her right side and also around her scapula. Again her neck muscles on both sides were tight and quite painful. During the treatment I played some relaxing music and suggested Mrs M try to imagine she was in her favourite place. Mrs M enjoyed her massage although she had felt some muscles were sensitive at first upon massaging. She really felt the benefit of the massage, felt re-energized and that a lot of her tension had disappeared.

Third visit: two weeks later

Mrs M commented that her back, neck and shoulders had not been as tense as usual. Her husband had also commented to her that he had found her not so 'crabby' and was more enjoyable to be around.

For this treatment I recommended a full body massage as Mrs M had again been busy and was feeling tense and tired. It also gave me a chance to do some work on her arms, wrists and hands. I found her arms to be very congested and as her arthritis in her hands had flared up, I did some gentle active and resisted exercises.

I advised Mrs M to come back to have some more massage on her arms, as I did not have enough time to work on them during a full body massage. After her massage Mrs M felt pampered, said she had not felt so relaxed in ages and left floating on air.

Fourth visit: one week later

Mrs M commented on a decrease in the number of headaches she had been having and that she had slept very well the night after her last treatment. However, she was still experiencing some pain in her wrists and in her forearms.

I massaged Mrs M's arms for half and hour to get rid of the congestion, to improve drainage and to ease any muscle spasm. It was also beneficial for her hands and fingers too in that it helped improve her joint mobility.

Outcome

Following massage Mrs M found she could cope better with her stress and her workload and had more energy. Her tension and the aching in her muscles disappeared with regular massage as did her headaches. She now also knew about the benefits of massage therapy and knew that if her signs and symptoms of stress returned all she had to do was to make another appointment. She would also still come once a month for an MOT session. We agreed that this would help all aspects of her life as massage also boosts the immune system.

Additional techniques and therapies

Alexander technique

The Alexander technique is a form of 'body work' therapy. Introduced by Australian, Fredrick Alexander in the late 1800s the technique focuses on posture and body movement as a key to good health and well-being. The premise that we often have poor posture while undertaking routine daily tasks such as sitting, standing, walking, etc., led to the technique's focus on conscious change in posture. An Alexander technique teacher will observe whole movement patterns and advise on aspects of individual patterns that may lead to problems. A range of conditions have been suggested as benefiting from the Alexander technique including back and neck pain and respiratory disorders. This technique teaches the individual how to change movement and posture patterns to reduce pressure on the body.

Case study: The Alexander technique
By Margaret Rakusen

Lisa was 48 years old and came to me for an introductory session in early December 2000. She had decided to try the Alexander technique to see if it would help her ongoing back problem.

Lisa had been having pain and discomfort in her back for approximately 15 years. Her lower back was very painful. She would get sharp pains from it at night that woke her up, and was in fairly continuous pain during the day. A canoeing accident seven years previously had led to neck problems which she still suffered from, although she had been for physiotherapy at the time which had eased it somewhat. However, the problems returned and her neck was always prone to stiffness.

I explained to her that in the Alexander technique we would be looking at the way in which she was carrying out her daily activities and that I would teach her the best way of doing these, so that she would no longer damage herself. I noticed that she held her head in an attitude that was causing a lot of very harmful pressures on her spine and discs.

Lisa decided to come for a course of 20–30 lessons with seven lessons fairly close together at the beginning so that we could get some improvements fairly quickly. After that she would come for weekly sessions, changing to fortnightly when she was ready to attend less often.

Lisa began her lessons and soon started to improve. In the lessons I showed her a different way of sitting, standing, walking, writing, lying down and how to turn her head without damaging her neck. We also looked at ways of improving her breathing and how to bend and lift without any strain. Lisa applied everything I taught her when she was carrying out her everyday activities and soon built up confidence in her ability to move freely without triggering her back problems. She told me that on occasions when she forgot and her back gave warning twinges she was able to quickly put everything right because she knew what was causing the problem. This has given Lisa confidence in her own ability to look after herself.

Conclusion: two months later
Lisa continued to make steady progress and attended fortnightly. Her neck was much less stiff and her lower back no longer gave her the continuous pain during the day or the sharp pains at night. She had recently completed a 10 mile walk without any painful after-effects.

Bowen therapy
by Catherine Vivian

Nature of Bowen therapy
Bowen therapy is a new and unique holistic therapy. It has been available in the UK since the early 1990s and was developed in Australia in the second half of the 20th century by Tom Bowen who gave it its name. The therapist performs a series of very gentle but specific moves of rolling skin over tissue, which are done at exact points on the body and in a particular sequence. This promotes the body's own healing responses through stimulation of nerve reflexes through muscle tissue and fascia. The whole connective tissue system is stimulated through increased lymphatic activity, and venous and arterial blood flow. As a result, the structural integrity of the body is improved, which in turn promotes overall health.

A number of theories have been put forward as to how this is achieved. Michael Nixon-Livy (1999) who has pioneered another form of Bowen therapy called the neurostructural integration technique known as NST said,

> 'The body is a self-regulating and bioenergetic phenomenon ... Tom Bowen realized that the body would regulate itself and return to balance if the appropriate neurological and neuromuscular context was created.

A number of varying techniques of Bowen therapy are developing. The most widely known is a 'light touch' therapy called the Bowen technique based on the original work of Tom Bowen. Other types of Bowen therapy have been developed all over the world from the original therapy, or taking their foundation from Bowen's later work. Some of these are: fascial kinetics (International School of Bowen Therapy), myopractic, neural touch, neurofascial massage (NFM) Bowen, SMART Bowen (advocated by Brian Smart, involving the Bowen technique plus NST and vibromuscular harmonization technique).

There exists considerable anecdotal evidence that Bowen therapy has a wide application and has helped people with conditions ranging from musculo-skeletal complaints, sports injuries, chronic pain, asthma, migraine, sleep quality, psychological conditions, cerebral palsy, attention deficit hyperactive disorder (ADHD), autism, etc. Whitaker (1997) has shown that the therapy positively affects heart rate, which is a measure of the functioning of the autonomic nervous system. The first academic study of a Bowen therapy in the UK was peformed by Bernie Carter, Professor of Children's Nursing at the University of Central Lancashire on clients' experiences of frozen shoulder (Carter, 2001).

The Bowen move

The Bowen move is quite specific in its lightness of pressure, slow speed of application, and position on the body where it is applied. Experienced practitioners develop sensitivity to the level of tension in the tissue, which tells them how to apply the move for optimum effect. With experience they can pinpoint the exact spot where it is needed.

In preparation the practitioner stands at one side of the patient who is lying prone. The practitioner locates the muscle that lies immediately to the side of the spine approximately 2.5 cm above the crest of the ileum. The thumb is placed on the belly of the muscle. There should be enough contact pressure to then take up any slack in the skin by drawing it back towards the practitioner, over the tissue until it is taut. At this point the thumb is up against the lateral side of the muscle allowing a light pressure to challenge it and make it stand slightly proud. The move is also done over ligaments and tendons in a similar fashion.

A gentle, slow roll of the skin is performed towards the spine (medially) over the tissue. The thumb maintains contact with the surface skin layer but allows the skin to roll over the tissue below. The pressure is not enough to force a painful stretch of the muscle, but strong enough to exert a change in local tissue tension. According to Wilks (2004) the action of this type of move elicits a powerful effect on the body on a number of levels, not just the musculo-skeletal system.

Changes are now set in motion more widely in the body due to stimulation of the neurovascular bundles in the tissue close to the move. The effects can be focused in particular areas by a move providing interference in tissue tension which produces an energy block, around which other moves can then be applied. The practitioner allows changes to take effect for a few minutes before applying the next set of moves (known as a procedure). The practitioner may even leave the room during this time to enable the patient to relax more deeply which can help the treatment.

Case studies: Bowen therapy
by Catherine Vivian

Case Study 1
Anna (name changed) is a delightful intelligent little girl aged 6 years who has mild quadriplegic cerebral palsy. Her main problem areas are with co-ordination, low muscle tone, balance, and walking. She has splints on both legs, uses sticks most of the time and a wheelchair for long distances.

Following Bowen therapy Anna's parents felt they saw definite improvements in her co-ordination so helping her overall balance. Her side-stepping and stepping backwards was better and she appeared to be standing up straighter. This had improved her confidence. Anna's hip muscles were tight before the treatment. They did ease up and she found it easier to flex the hip and bend the leg upwards. Her walking is slower, more controlled and with a better heel-to-toe action. She is also able to walk for longer periods. Anna continues to have regular treatments.

Case study 2
Charlie (name changed) is a 9-year-old boy with hypotonic cerebral palsy who had a difficult birth. He has problems in many areas, with profound hearing loss and no speech. As a lively little boy, he moves around mostly on his bottom, having difficulty walking, but loves to climb around everything. He is unable to chew and has problems with liquids. Family life is hard as his behaviour is loud, demanding and very physical with a lot of biting and scratching. His tolerance of being handled is low with a fierce temper and he easily becomes agitated. His parents said this had got worse as he became more mobile. His sleeping pattern was never good, he often wakes around 3 a.m. and disturbs the whole house with his noise.

After the first Bowen treatment session Charlie's parents noticed immediate changes. He slept soundly that night from 9 p.m. to 7 a.m., and his Dad carried him downstairs without the usual biting and scratching. The second most marked improvement was in his behaviour, with fewer tantrums and significantly less violence. Tantrums became quicker to overcome as communicating with him was easier. Eye contact improved and he was watching Maketon signing a lot more. His parents felt that his concentration and attention levels had changed for the better. His elder sister also noticed this when she played games with him. She said his sensitivity to noises had increased, and his concentration when playing with toys was longer. His laughter had changed from a throaty giggle to a deep belly laugh that left him breathless.

Charlie's normal babbling now included some clearly enunciated sounds such as the letter 'r'. Feeding had improved slightly with less choking, and he was spoon-feeding himself more with better control of the spoon. Mobility, co-ordination and balance showed slight improvements. His climbing and shuffling movements were undertaken with more apparent skill. Charlie has continued having Bowen therapy and has since shown even more radical improvements in a number of areas. As a consequence the life of the family has changed significantly for the better.

References

Borotoft J (1996) Massage for mental health *Therapist* **4**(1): 38–44.

Burns A, Byrne J, Ballard C, Holmes C (2002) Sensory stimulation in dementia. *Br Med J* **325**:1312–13.

Carter B (2001) A pilot study to evaluate the effectiveness of Bowen Technique in the management of clients with frozen shoulder. *Complementary Therapies in Nursing* **9**(4): 208.

Edge J (2003) A pilot study addressing the effect of aromatherapy massage on mood, anxiety and relaxation in adult mental health. *Complementary Therapies in Nursing and Midwifery* **9**: 90–7.

Ferrell-Torry A, Glick O (1993) The use of therapeutic massage as a nursing intervention to modify anxiety and the perception of cancer pain. *Cancer Nursing* **16**: 93–101.

Field T, Morrow C, Valedon C, Larson S, Kuhn C, Schanberg S (1993) Massage reduces anxiety in child and adolescent psychiatric patients. *International Journal of Alternative Complementary Medicine* **11**(7): 22–7.

Flemming K (1997) The meaning of hope to palliative care cancer patients. *International Journal of Palliative Nursing* **3**:14–18.

Gray R (2000) The use of massage therapy in palliative care. *Complementary Therapies in Nursing and Midwifery* **6**: 77–82.

Jelinek A, Novakora B (2001) The psychotherapeutic use of essential oils. *International Journal of Aromatherapy* **11**(2): 100–2.

Joyce M, Richardson R (1997) Reflexology can help MS. *International Journal of Alternative and Complementary Medicine* **July**: 10–12.

Kohn M (2000) *Complementary Therapies in Cancer Care*. London: Macmillan Cancer Relief.

Maxwell Hudson C (1996) *The Complete Book of Massage*. London: Dorling Kindersley.

Nixon-Livy M (1999) Neurostructural Integration Technique – Advanced Bowen Therapy. *Positive Health Magazine*, August.

Peters D, Chaitlow L, Harris G, Morrison S (2002) *Integrating Complementary Therapies in Primary Care*. Edinburgh: Churchill Livingstone.

Preece J (2002) Introducing abdominal massage in palliative care for the relief of constipation. *Complementary Therapies in Nursing and Midwifery* **8**: 101–5.

Rankin Box D (ed) (2001) *The Nurses Handbook of Complementary Therapies*. London: Bailliere Tindall.

Tiran D (1996) The use of complementary therapies in midwifery practice a focus on reflexology. *Complementary Therapies in Nursing and Midwifery* **2**(2): 32–7.

Whitaker JA (1997) *The Bowen Technique, a Gentle Hands-on Healing Method that Affects the Autonomic Nervous System, as Measured by Heart Rate Variability and Clinical Assessment*. Paper presented to the American Academy of Environmental Medicine at La Jolla, CA, USA.

Wilks J (2004) *Understanding the Bowen Technique*. Gloucester: First Stone Publishing in association with the Bowen Therapy Academy of Australia and the Bowen Association of the UK.

Woolfson A, Hewitt D (1992) Intensive aromacare. *International Journal of Aromatherapy* **4**(2): 12–13.

Wright S, Courtney U, Donnelly C, Kenny T, Lavin C (2002) Clients' perceptions of the benefits of reflexology on their quality of life. *Complementary Therapies in Nursing and Midwifery* **8**: 69–76.

Further reading and sources of information

Aromatherapy
www.aromatherapy-regulation.org.uk

Bach flower remedies
www.bachcentre.com

Massage
Sayre-Adams J, Wright SG (2001) *Therapeutic Touch*. London: Harcourt.

www.gcmt.org.uk

www.cmhmassage.co.uk

Infant massage
Simpson R (2001) Baby Massage classes and the work of the International Association of Infant Massage. *Complementary Therapies in Nursing and Midwifery* **7**: 25–33.

www.iaim.org.uk

Reflexology

Williamson J (1999) *A Guide to Precision Reflexology*. London: Mark Allen Publishing.

www.reflexologyforum.org

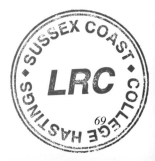

Chapter 6

_____

Therapies in focus:
Reiki, counselling, hypnotherapy, meditation, crystal therapy and yoga

Reiki

Any discussion around reiki must begin with an explanation of the eastern view of 'universal energy'. This notion of a form of energy within all living organisms underpins many of the therapies and systems of medicine stemming from the east. Energy work has a long history. We have moved from a reductionist view of the body and its systems to a view that the body interacts with the environment.

The concept of life energy in the West has been influenced by world perspectives including Indian and Chinese. The notion of a vital life force is a key component of the belief systems of these cultures but in the West we often have difficulty in translating this concept.

In India, prana is the concept of a life force that exists within and around every living being. In China this is known as chi. Many complementary therapies use the principles of human life force in the healing processes. For example, within Chinese medicine the balance of chi is vitally important to health. Where chi is abundant and flowing freely through the body good health will remain. However, where the flow of chi is blocked, disease may occur.

Reiki (pronounced ray – key) is a healing technique that involves the 'laying on of hands'. Reiki is a Japanese word with rei meaning universal and ki meaning life force. The interpretation of these terms within Japanese culture is much more complex. However, in the West we have taken these two words to describe this form of healing.

Reiki is not a religion or affiliated with any religion. It uses the universal life force to assist the body's natural defences to heal itself. In good health the life force energy (ki) flows freely round the body through vessels or channels and is also found outside of the body within a field called the aura. When the energy flow is blocked the body can be affected negatively and ill health may occur. Traditional reiki began in the mid-1800s with Mikao Usui who led the teaching on reiki through Japan. This teaching was then brought to the West via America The teaching of reiki is passed from a reiki master to student with the most common teaching being split into three levels – 1, 2 and master level. The teaching technique uses an attunement whereby the student becomes a 'channel' for healing energy. From this point the healer will be able to consciously 'request' the energy to flow. It is the attunement process that sets reiki apart from other 'hands on' healing. The attunement creates the healer; it opens channels for healing. During the first month after attunement the healer has to adjust to this energy flow and may experience a number of symptoms of detoxification. At this level the student learns hand positions and the procedure to follow prior to, during and after healing.

Level 2 teaches different techniques for healing with further attunement to strengthen the healing power. At this level the reiki student learns distant healing and this level also stimulates and strengthens institution. Most reiki teachers agree that there should be at least a month between levels 1 and 2.

At the third level the student who wishes to become a reiki master will often wait months or even years to take this next step. A reiki master will often teach others or may just use this level for healing. This level of reiki requires dedication and responsibility as attunement to the highest level brings a lifetime commitment to healing.

During a treatment the receiver of reiki remains fully clothed and the practitioner will use specific hand positions on the body to channel healing energy. During the 1980s independent research by Becker and Zimmerman investigated the nature of therapies like reiki and looked at its impact on the physiology of the body. During this study they found that the brain waves of the practitioner and healer became synchronized in the alpha state, which is characteristic of deep relaxation, and the biomagnetic field of the practitioner's hands is 100 times greater than normal. It is also suggested that the practitioner and receiver resonate in unison with the earth's magnetic field. This is known as the Schumann resonance; the practitioner and receiver link with the earth's energy field via the Schumann resonance. It is suggested in further studies that it is the frequency at which this biomagnetic field pulsates that stimulates healing (Steine and Steine, 2003).

Organization and regulation

The UK has a number of established organizations to support reiki practitioners and to maintain the highest standards of practice. The Reiki Regulatory Working Group works with organizations who promote voluntary self-regulation, have a code of ethics, standards of practice and a disciplinary procedure. The group has also been involved in developing national occupational standards.

Reiki within health care

Reiki is experiencing growing popularity and within health care in the UK it is the subject of conference discussions and journal papers. Publications from the

US highlight studies within acute and palliative care of the use of reiki within the health care system (Rankin Box, 2003). However, the findings may not be considered conclusive due to the nature of the limitations of these studies. This is a common feature within research around these types of therapies and often we are left with anecdotal evidence. The following case study highlights an example of a specific health condition that has been treated using reiki in the UK.

Case study: Reiki
by Jackie Wiles

Marjorie is a lady in her late 70s who has osteoarthritis in her hips and knees. Her consultant had recently told her that surgery was not an option in her case as she had such a degree of heart failure that a general anaesthetic would be too risky. She had always been a very active woman and the prospect of becoming crippled by arthritis was very distressing to her. Her treatment was centred on simply controlling the pain and Marjorie was very unhappy about this. Marjorie was introduced to me by a friend of mine and I agreed to see her for an hour a week.

When I first met Marjorie, she was pale, weak, breathless and very depressed. She told me that the pain in her knees was causing her a lot of discomfort and the analgesia that her consultant had prescribed was not really controlling her pain. Her mobility was rapidly deteriorating and she was finding normal daily activities very difficult. She was desperate for some relief from the pain and stiffness caused by her arthritis.

Reiki energy directs itself to the areas of greatest need and after the first session, there was no real improvement in her arthritis but a noticeable improvement in her symptoms of heart failure. During the second session the pain in her knees was temporarily increased as the energy seemed to direct itself to her joints. By the time she came for the third session she was walking well, there were no obvious signs of heart failure and her psychological state was very positive.

Over the next few weeks, her general health continued to improve, as did her mobility. Her pain has become less in general but she still has some 'bad days' and she has had some relapses. However, the general trend has been towards an improvement in her condition. In fact there has been such an improvement in Marjorie's general health that she has now been referred back to her consultant who has agreed to reconsider surgery.

I would not say that reiki has cured her arthritis but it has made it more manageable. What was most noticeable to me was the improvement in her psychological state. She is no longer depressed and she has stopped worrying about the future and begun living more in the present. She is now much more accepting of her condition and able to cope with the changes that arthritis has made to her daily life.

As both a nurse and reiki practitioner, I would like to see reiki being used in conjunction with medicine as a complementary treatment. Reiki helps the body to reach its own natural balance, which optimizes the ability to recover from ill health. Working alongside modern medicine reiki could speed recovery times and help to maintain health after a major illness or surgery. In cases where full recovery is not possible reiki could help patients come to terms with life-changing events, such as in mastectomy or amputations.

'Talking therapies'

The therapies grouped here have often been termed the 'talking therapies'. These therapies include counselling, psychotherapy and neurolinguistic programming (NLP). Life coaching may also be included.

These therapies are identified with psychological support for the patient but it is the mind–body link that can be used as a focus within complementary therapies. Many of the physiological effects of stress are acknowledged, including hypertension, irritable bowel and a range of conditions thought to have a psychological link. The notion that health is more than just physical health also helps us to understand the importance of psychological well-being in determining health.

For some, counselling is required a particular times in their lives, for example, following a bereavement, for others counselling may be required to help them to deal with long-term health problems or may be seen as a tool to prevent ill health. There are a number of different types of counselling and counselling based on different schools of thought.

Approaches may include person-centred counselling, bereavement counselling and psychotherapeutic counselling. Some counselling approaches may focus on different aspects of the problem while other approaches may deal specifically with one issue, i.e. bereavement.

Types of counselling

There are several types of counselling. Each has its own theory and its own way of working. Some practitioners draw on elements of several different models when working with clients.

For the client an important factor is whether the counsellor is directive (where the client is given suggested courses of action and activities to do outside of the session) or non-directive (where the client takes the lead in what is discussed).

The following are some of the counselling approaches most commonly used.

- *Client-centred or person-centred counselling*: This approach uses the relationship with the counsellor to create particular therapeutic conditions These are: empathy, unconditional positive regard and congruence. This approach is often used with emotional issues such as bereavement to allow feelings to be worked through.
- *Psychodynamic counselling*: This approach is based on the view that past experiences have an effect on experiences and feelings in the present, and that important relationships, perhaps from early childhood, may be replayed with other people later in life. Developing a trusting and reliable relationship with the counsellor is essential for this work as the counsellor remains neutral to ensure that the client can be as open about past relationships as possible.
- *Transpersonal counselling*: Transpersonal counselling places the emphasis on personal empowerment. The underpinning belief in this approach is that although we may suffer a number of hardships in our life experience the core of the individual remains unchanged and this can be worked with. It takes account of the client's past experiences, but also looks to the future, acknowledging some of the qualities the individual will need to use to meet those challenges.
- *Cognitive-behavioural counselling*: This is a directive model, The objective of this approach is to change self-defeating or irrational beliefs and behaviours by altering negative ways of thinking. The approach encourages the individual to monitor his or her own feelings, thoughts and behaviours and to identify and challenge those which may need challenging. This is an active approach where counsellors usually give clients tasks or homework to do between sessions. This could mean recording thoughts and feelings, or doing something that tests out a basic assumption about themselves.

Other approaches to counselling may include:

- Transactional analysis counselling.
- Existential counselling.
- Personal construct counselling.
- Gestalt counselling.
- Rational-emotive behavioural counselling.

Neurolingistic programming (NLP) has a particular focus on how we use language to create particular thought processes. Work within NLP helps the person to explore how they feel about a problem or issue and then look at ways in which unwanted habits and behaviours can be changed. This focus helps people to view an issue in a more positive way or to unblock some of the negative thoughts they may hold.

Psychological therapies such as counselling and NLP all seek to assist the individual to find an alternative to the unwanted behaviours, feelings and thoughts. They tend to act generally with the conscious mind (NLP works between conscious and unconscious mind). Hypnotherapy is different in that its focus is on promoting this change, working with the unconscious mind.

Hypnotherapy
by Tom Tait

Historical perspective

The concept of using trances to alleviate illness recurs throughout the history of medicine. Over 4000 years ago one of the founders of Asian medicine Wang Tai used words as a healing tool, and hieroglyphics on Egyptian tombs from 3000 BC record a form of hypnosis. The oldest written record of hypnotic cures was obtained from Ebers Paparys which described practices used in Egyptian medicine before 1552 BC. This describes a physician placing hands on the head of the patient and claiming superhuman therapeutic powers giving forth strange utterances or suggestions which resulted in cure. Hippocrates, the Greek physician often referred to as the 'father of medicine', is also known to have discussed the phenomenon.

Modern hypnotherapy commenced in the 18th century when a flamboyant Austrian physician named Franz Mesmer arrived in Paris and went on to develop the theory of 'animal magnetism'. He faced many critics who accused him of being a charlatan but today Mesmer is regarded as a pioneer in the development of hypnotism and psychotherapy.

A hypnotherapy session normally contains a number of stages – eye closure, progressive relaxation, visualizations, deepeners and, with some treatments, post-hypnotic suggestions. The induction is a ritual that the hypnotherapist employs to achieve progressive relaxation of the body and mind to reach a state of hyper-suggestibility often referred to as a trance. Many procedures can be employed by a skilled hypnotherapist to achieve the patient's detachment from his or her surroundings.

A common approach is talking quietly and making repeated suggestions that the client is becoming increasingly relaxed and the eyelids are becoming heavy. Other approaches include asking the client to look at a spinning disk and count slowly backwards from 30 to zero. As clients slip into a trance they will feel very relaxed. The conscious mind will no longer control every thought as it does when an individual is awake. The surroundings will become less important and clients become increasingly aware of their feelings and sensations. During a session the sense of time will become distorted and clients will find it hard to calculate how long they have been in a trance.

To encourage patients to reach a deeper level of trance the hypnotherapist will employ a deepening technique. Again repetitions are used such as, 'You are going deeper and deeper', and you are asked to visualize scenes or experiences you find peaceful and relaxing. Interestingly, the deepness of the trance in relation to the effectiveness of treatment has become an area of academic debate. In other words there does not appear to be a consensus in the profession as to the correlation between depth of trance and success of treatments.

In conclusion hypnotherapy is now accepted as a legitimate treatment for fears, phobias and other associated disorders. However, it is not an appropriate therapy for physical problems that require a medical diagnosis. It is also not usable in certain serious psychological problems such as psychosis and endogenous depression.

Uses within health care

A number of conditions have been noted by Ernst (2001) as benefiting from hypnotherapy. These include:

- Stress.
- Anxiety.
- Phobias.
- Addiction.
- Depression.
- Irritable bowel syndrome.
- Asthma.

Hypnotherapy may also be used to prepare for medical treatment or within dentistry.

Training, education and regulation

Specific training or regulation is not required by law at present. A number of professional associations keep registers of practitioners and the General Hypnotherapy Standards Council keeps the General Hypnotherapy Register. The British Society of Medical and Dental Hypnosis (BSMDH) is a group of health practitioners who practise hypnotherapy.

Case study: Hypnotherapy
by Tom Tait

Case study 1
Sheila, aged 24, had suffered a bad job interview experience where she had found herself feeling shaky and talking too much and too fast. Needless to say, this behaviour had halted her career advancement. She also said that the more people there were on the interview panel the more nervous she was. Sheila made an appointment to see a clinical hypnotherapist who used relaxation and visualization techniques to teach her to relax before an interview. Under trance Sheila was advised to visualize the feelings she would have when she was congratulated on being appointed. She displayed a surge of elation as positive feelings flowed through her body.

Just before going into her interview she was instructed to recall the trance experience and visualize getting the job. The visualization became a self-fulfilling prophecy. She performed at interview in a more relaxed way and displayed remarkable confidence. She was offered the job.

Case study 2
Margaret, aged 45, was a traffic warden who had been smoking 30 cigarettes per day for 20 years. She wished to give up smoking but found it hard to do so with a number of failed attempts behind her. Under hypnosis Julie was given the suggestion that she could feel calm and relaxed without cigarettes, that she would hate the smell of cigarette smoke and she would find the whole idea of cigarette smoking abhorrent. She was given repeated suggestions that she could feel calm and relaxed without a cigarette, planting enough positive ideas into her subconscious mind to create the desired motivation for change. Margaret is now a natural non-smoker some 18 months after her treatment.

Case study 3
Bob, aged 50, ran a small general store. The job involved long hours and whenever he felt bored or irritable he turned to his limitless supply of crisps or sweets. He used food like a drug to lift his mood and no longer responded to his body's natural feelings of hunger. Over three years he had put on 20 kg. He had tried lots of different diets and had lost some weight but as soon as he stopped dieting, he put the weight back on. This inability to control his weight made him depressed.

Under hypnosis Bob was given powerful suggestions that he should use food to maintain his body in good health, that he would develop control over his eating and have regular meals in response to his hunger. He would stop eating the moment he felt full and would not like junk food. He was also told he would focus on being more calm and relaxed.

Bob had four sessions of clinical hypnosis. During this time his weight started to drop. Listening to his body's cues of hunger, planning healthy meals and sitting down with his family at set times to eat dinner, Bob lost an average of 1.2 kg per week and reached his target weight in just over a year.

Meditation

Meditation has been used for centuries within many cultures. The practice of meditation has been described within Christianity, Buddhism, Hinduism, Islam, Taoism, Shinto and the pagan and shamanistic belief systems. In the West meditation was particularly used in the Russian and Greek orthodox churches with repetition of a 'mantra', usually the Jesus Prayer, being the most common form of meditative process. Although these religions and belief systems have used meditation, contemplation and prayer, meditation does not require any allegiance to any belief system.

Meditation is the ability to quieten the mind and focus thoughts inwards. through relaxed concentration upon a chosen stimulus. For some this may include the chanting of a particular phrase or word known as a mantra, for others the stimulus may be a candle, crystal or a picture. Focusing on this chosen stimulus allows the distractions usually present within the mind to be pushed to one side. Meditation does, however, take practice but once mastered this concentration can be practised on a busy train or in a crowded room.

The benefits of meditation

Deep relaxation has been described as having a number of health benefits including a reduction in blood pressure, improved posture as the mind focuses on the position of the body, and, for some, better pain management. Chapter 7 includes a contribution from a practising nurse using visualization for pain management in children.

Crystal therapy

Identified within the House of Lords Select Committee Report (Department of Health, 2001) as a recognized therapy but one that lacks a substantial evidence base crystal healing is used by many people who hold beliefs about the benefits of energy healing.

What is it?

Throughout history crystals and gemstones have been surrounded in myth and mystery. Linked to healing and spirituality, crystals were used by ancient Egyptian priests and rulers, with gemstone-lined headdresses and amethyst found in the tombs of pharaohs. In ancient Rome wine was often served in amethyst cups as this was seen to protect the drinker from 'drunkenness'. There is also the well-known connection between the 'tellers of fortunes' and crystal balls. However, within this myth and magic a scientific paradigm exists. Natural crystals contain too many flaws for precision use, and within technology synthesized crystals of silicon are used to create silicon chips for use in computers, etc. Many crystals created in the laboratory keep the same atomic structure as their natural counterparts but are developed synthetically to avoid flaws. The quartz crystal is the cornerstone of modern day measurement of time. Piezoelectric vibrations from quartz crystal are used to run watches, computers, televisions and a range of everyday appliances. This piezoelectric activity creates a tiny electrical charge when pressure is applied to a specific crystal and crystals vary in their structure and electromagnetic field. Crystalline structures exist within the body on the surface of our cells and in the mitochondria. It is this that links the power of crystals to healing.

How does it work?

Crystal healing uses gemstones and minerals in a holistic approach aimed at improving a person's health on all levels. On an emotional level crystals have the capacity to heal specific emotional states and on a physiological level it is suggested that when a crystal is used in therapy and placed near to nerve clusters this will alter the behaviour of the neurotransmitter messengers and therefore alter body chemistry. Balance in the energy field is achieved through vibration of specific crystals that match the vibrations of the individual's energy field. Crystals are chosen by the therapist to balance energy through the whole body system as well as using specific crystals for specific ailments. During a therapy session crystals may be placed on the clothed body at various points, usually those related to the chakras. Crystals may also be placed in the area around the body, in the energy field. Those people who use crystals for healing purposes will follow a ritual of cleansing the crystals to reduce negative energy absorbed by the crystal during the healing process.

Using crystals

Ten of most common crystals used in healing are:

- *Clear quartz* (transparent): A versatile crystal thought to ampify other crystals, aids meditation.

- *Rose quartz* (pink): A member of the quartz family, rose quartz has an infinity with emotions of love and is often linked to the heart. It is seen as a soothing crystal and is particularly good for children.
- *Amethyst* (from pale lavender to deep violet): This crystal promotes spiritual awareness, it is calming and good for headaches when placed on the forehead. Excellent for meditation.
- *Carnelian* (translucent reddish brown): This crystal is used for blood disorders, and it reduces anger and inflammation. Stimulating.
- *Lapis lazuli* (blue): This crystal is protective. It protects against depression, boosts the immune system and aids self-expression.
- *Aventurine quartz* (yellow/brown to bluish green): This is a general healing stone, it is stress relieving and soothing.
- *Citrine* (pale green/yellow): This crystal is cleansing and promotes emotional maturity, it is used in digestive problems. It attracts abundance.
- *Malachite* (green, often with banding): This crystal is soothing and calming. It is excellent for meditation and amplifies current mood.
- *Hematite* (dark grey to black with a metallic sheen): Historically, this crystal was linked to the blood, thought to be due to its iron oxide content. It is a grounding stone that is very useful for transforming negativity.
- *Tiger's eye* (black to dark brown with yellow and golden banding): This crystal develops inner strength, protects from eye disease and enhances creativity.

Uses of crystal healing within health care

Currently this therapy is not widely used in health care. However, in common with a number of energy healing therapies, many of our patients/clients may access these therapies to complement their orthodox treatment or may seek information about them. It is therefore important that health care practitioners are able to give appropriate information or guide patients to appropriate resources.

Training, education and regulation

Crystal healing therapists may undergo specific training in this therapy in a range of courses from workshops through to diploma courses. Therapists may also register with one of the recognized organizations in the UK, including the International Association of Crystal Healing Therapists and the Affiliation of Crystal Healing Organizations. At present there is no single body for regulation and self-regulation has developed.

Yoga

What is yoga?

Yoga is an ancient Indian practice using physical postures to obtain a harmony of mind, body and spirit. Yoga has existed for centuries and has been used by many cultures in the East. From its roots in Eastern culture yoga was bought to Europe in the 1800s by those returning from residence in colonial India, and grew in popularity in the West over time during the 20th century. The British Wheel of Yoga founded in the 1960s was the first yoga organization in Britain. Yoga's growing popularity came at a time when many people where becoming interested in the link between mind and body and the notion of holism.

The word yoga comes from Sanskrit, the ancient language of India, meaning oneness. Meditation is a key feature as the control of body and mind is central to yoga.

In the West, yoga is often seen as just another form of exercise. There are many forms of yoga including the following:

- *Astanga* is a set sequence of postures that will not vary from class to class. The sequence will move through a primary, secondary, and then advanced series, the aim of which is to leave you feeling energized and balanced with an inner alertness. It is not a beginner's method as some knowledge of postures and their correct form is required.
- *Bikram* is a form of yoga that teaches 26 postures in a set sequence in a room heated to about 38°C. It is suitable for both beginners or advanced students as the same pattern is always followed. The aim of the class is mostly physical improvement, although internal cleansing will also take place.
- *Hatha* is the basis of most yoga classes. Hatha has its roots in the ancient systems first documented over 2000 years ago. Its aim is to balance you both physically and mentally and will leave you feeling both stimulated and relaxed. It is suitable for both beginners and more advanced students, and classes will vary from teacher to teacher.
- *Iyengar* is a very thorough form of yoga that pays attention to detail. The emphasis during a class is on correct alignment. The class is very suitable for beginners as it helps to learn each asana. The concentration involved in perfecting technique also helps to focus the mind.
- *Kundalini* is perhaps the most spiritual of all the yoga disciplines. Kundalini combines asanas with mudras, mantras and breathing to allow connection with the chakras.
- *Power yoga.* Similar to astanga yoga, this form was recently developed in America to offer a tough cardio workout.

- *Sivananda*. This form may use mantras and meditation. It is based on 12 basic hatha postures and has a strong emphasis on breathing technique. Much of a class will also be devoted to relaxation. You will be left feeling uplifted and mentally focused.
- *Viniyoga* is a specific one-to-one form of yoga that aims to address an individual's needs, both mental and physical.

Hatha yoga is the form of yoga most used in the West and connected with exercise, however this form of yoga also attempts to consolidate mind, body and energy flow. Yoga practices, such as stretching, correct posture, deep breathing, meditation and visualization, can all prevent the negative effects of stress. It is this aspect of yoga that is its attraction for many practitioners. Hatha yoga consists largely of practising the asana or positions. The asana aim to free the body's flow of energy in a controlled way. The role of controlled breathing in reducing blood pressure and therefore stress levels is well documented. Additionally, yoga therapists suggest that the following health benefits can be gained from yoga:

- Increased oxygenation of the blood.
- Muscle toning throughout the body.
- Clearer and more relaxed mind.
- Improved posture.
- Improved circulation of blood and lymph.
- Regulation of bodily functions.

With this in mind it is possible to see the implications for health care.

Implications for health care

Yoga therapy involves the use of yoga to improve and/or maintain health. Research evidence shows that yoga may help conditions including asthma, hypertension and joint mobility (Ernst, 2001). It is also suggested that mild depression may be helped with yoga (Woolery et al, 2004). Yoga therapy may be a useful addition to rehabilitation for a number of different health conditions.

Training, education and regulation

At present there is no single body for the regulation of yoga practitioners and no defined course curriculum. Practitioners may belong to one of a number of organizations and these are working with the British Council for Yoga Therapy to develop a single register and standards for training.

References

Department of Health (2001) *Government Response to the House of Lords Select Committee on Science and Technology's Report on Complementary and Alternative Medicine.* London: Department of Health.

Ernst E (2001) *The Desktop Guide to Complementary Medicine.* St Louis: Mosby

Rankin-Box (Ed) (2001) *The Nurses Book of Complementary Therapies* (2nd Edn.) London: Bailliere and Tindall.

Steine B, Steine F (2003) The Reiki Source Book. London, Oriental Press.

Further reading and sources of information

Crystal therapy

Hall J (2003) *The Crystal Bible.* Llandeilo, Wales: Cygnus Books.

Simpson L (1997) *The Book of Crystal Healing.* London: Gaia.

Hypnotherapy

British Society of Medical and Dental Hypnosis (BSMDH). www.bsmdh.org

General Hypnotherapy Standards Counci. www.ghsc.co.uk

Meditation

Fontana D (1998) *Learn to Meditate: The Art of Tranquillity Self-Awareness and Insight.* London: Duncan Baird Publishers

Reiki

Stein D (1995) *Essential Reiki: A Complete Guide to an Ancient Healing Art.* Berkeley, CA: Crossing Press.

Steine B, Steine F (2003) *The Reiki Source Book.* London: Oriental Press.

www.reikiregulation.org.uk

Yoga

Woolery A, Myers H, Sternlieb B, Zeltzer L (2004) A yoga intervention for young adults with elevated symptoms of depression. *Alternative Therapies in Health and Medicine* **10**(2): 60–3.

British Council for Yoga Therapy. www.yogatherapyforum.org.uk

Chapter 7

CAM therapies in practice:
Art therapy, music therapy and relaxation and imagery

The following are practising nurses' contributions to the work around particular complementary therapies including:

- Art therapy in the mental health setting.
- Music therapy in the theatre setting.
- Relaxation and imagery with children.

Art therapy in a mental health setting
by Zoe Murrell

According to Waller and Gilroy (1992: 5) art therapy is defined as

> *'A form of therapy in which the making of visual images (paintings, drawings, models, etc.) in the presence of a qualified art therapist contributes towards externalization of thoughts and feelings that may otherwise remain unexpressed'.*

It is acknowledged that for many years the investigation and interpretation of visual imagery and dreams have played an important role in gaining an insight into individual's deep-seated anxieties. Historically, imagery was acknowledged to be a powerful healing tool, which was used to enhance health through healing rituals and ceremonies. It is only in recent years that art therapy has been introduced as a profession, taking on board these concepts with the therapist receiving extensive training and having a comprehensive knowledge of various psychological theories (Waller, 1993).

The main aim of art therapy is for the therapist to assist the patient to explore and facilitate the release of emotion that might otherwise not have been openly and verbally communicated. Ultimately this type of therapy assists patients to work through their difficulties by exploring and unravelling the images they have created (Heywood, 2002). The images may have a diagnostic element as well as being creative, providing indicators of where further support is required (Thomson, 1997).

Individuals undertaking art therapy sessions may also be able to achieve personal growth, increase autonomy and confidence levels and help maintain a sense of their own identity. Others may simply choose to undertake art therapy sessions for exploration, motivation or enjoyment (Warren, 1993). Art therapy sessions must be undertaken within a safe, facilitative environment. Dalley (1984) goes on to state that, provided the environment is appropriate to the needs of the patient and the actual session, patients may begin to experience a sense of trust with their therapist. Many authors argue that trust is a key component when aiming to establish a therapeutic relationship with a patient. Trust involves sensitivity and illustrates professional skills that may enhance patients' confidence levels. Therefore the therapeutic relationship has to be based upon non-judgemental support, honesty, warmth and concern. If this can be established individuals may be more likely to achieve personal goals and ultimately begin to establish trust with others. A possible reason for this development of trust within art therapy may be due to these types of sessions offering an active rather than a passive role. Many clients may also remember a sense of play and creativity from their childhood, and may see this type of therapy as a means of fusing connections between childhood and present life (Heywood, 2002).

Working with clients with long-term mental illnesses, who have spent long periods of time within an institutional setting may find it difficult to engage in any form of one-to-one psychotherapy due to limited social skills and decreased confidence levels. The art room may provide freedom of choice and allow clients to express their feelings and thoughts directly through their artwork. They may be able to channel their emotions, both positive and negative, into their creations. This may provide an outlet for their thoughts and moods. Additionally, medication may not be able to touch on the depth and seriousness of a delusional system, whereas art therapy may initiate the unravelling of these difficulties. Art therapy may also offer the opportunity for individuals to move away from psychological suffering, as it can serve as an alternative view – allowing patients' concentration to be redirected. It is hoped that individuals will be focused on the art process, using materials and building the piece. In this way they may temporarily forget the psychological difficulties they are experiencing, thus relieving pain through distraction (Teasdale, 1988).

There is a plethora of art materials available that may be used within the art therapy session. These materials include crayons, watercolours, pastels, poster paints, paper and clay. The environment is also important; good lighting, a sink and a lockable storage area are necessary requirements (Heywood, 2002).

The main focus of art therapy is the actual image. This process involves a transaction between the creator (the patient), the artefact and the therapist.

Bringing unconscious feelings to a conscious level enables an exploration process to take place. Many authors believe that the richness of an artistic symbol and metaphor illuminates this process. Effective art therapists must have a considerable understanding of the art process and be proficient in non-verbal communication. They should also aim to provide a suitable environment (Kearney, 2000). The process of art therapy is based on the recognition that individuals' most fundamental thoughts and feelings, are derived from the unconscious mind and are expressed in images rather than words. Therefore the technique of art therapy is based on the knowledge that all individuals, whether trained or untrained, have a latent capacity to project their inner conflicts into a visual form. The emphasis then is on the images that arise from the patient's unconscious, which contains conflicts. The assumption is that once the conflicts are made concrete, they can be more easily understood by the patient and the therapist, which will in turn assist in their resolution (Schaverien, 1999).

There are several obstacles to facilitating art therapy within a mental health nursing setting. Cashell and Miner (1983) discovered worrying levels of fatigue and isolation among art therapists. This is because art therapists tend to work alone, rather than within a group, and therefore maintain the art therapy group sessions themselves, being unable to hand over or designate groups and sessions to other staff members. Stress may occur because the art therapist builds therapeutic relationships purely on a one-to-one basis, without assistance from the other health care staff. Moreover, it is reported that many art therapists have left the profession because of inadequate financial rewards and limited promotion prospects (Kearney, 2000).

There is also the problem of proving the effectiveness of, and need for, art therapy within a mental health setting to other health care professionals. This may be because art therapy is a relative newcomer to the world of therapeutic treatment, as opposed to psychology or social work (Schaverien, 1999). There is limited research into the effectiveness of art therapy as art therapists have little time or energy to carry out independent research, although some research has been undertaken by other health professionals. Because of this lack of empirical evidence to prove the efficacy of the therapy, many health care professionals are not fully aware of the usefulness of art therapy and consider that it simply does something vaguely helpful for patients (Warren, 1993).

Critics say that art therapy is helpful to patients only in that they are getting one-to-one sessions, and that the therapeutic benefits are not gained from the actual artwork created, or the interpretation of it (Teasdale, 1988). Another criticism is that different therapists may interpret drawings and paintings in different ways. Waller and Gilroy (1992) describe people 'making astonishing interpretations of peoples doodles'. Russell-Lacy (1979) does not see the relevance of art therapy, stating that there is no need for art therapy if the diagnosis has already been made.

'The art of schizophrenics does not display any particular unusual characteristics to warrant differential diagnosis through art.'

This appears to miss the point of art therapy, which is to facilitate a therapeutic relationship within which the patient can express emotions, fears and ideas and release pent up frustrations.

The use of complementary therapies may not only be beneficial to patients but also to nurses. If complementary therapies become incorporated into the working role of the nurse, this will enable the nurse to 'get back to the bedside' (Johnson, 2000) and to work more closely with the patient without having to rush, as time would be allowed for the intervention. Johnson (2000) also states, 'This is very positive as it suggests a way for nursing to move closer to achieving autonomy in practice...'

In conclusion, it is important to state that art therapy, while mostly concerned with addressing problems, is also about inspiring hope, strength and determination and about increasing confidence and motivation. It offers support at a time of emotional distress, a way of coming to terms with difficult and deep-seated anxieties, a safe place in which to express different kinds of feelings, and a means of improving communication. It offers an opportunity for the patient to play an active rather than a passive role. These advantages appear encouraging. However there are massive boundaries that need to be conquered in order for art therapy to gain a reputable following and an effective evidence base. Limited funding, training and available posts are still issues that prevent its widespread use. However, if these issues are addressed and acknowledged by the appropriate trusts and managers then art therapy could be incorporated into everyday nurse settings, become part of student nurses' core training and ultimately be used to create positive and holistic interactions with patients with mental illnesses, assisting them to be in more control of their deep-seated problems and anxieties. This would help to enable high quality patient outcomes.

Music therapy in a theatre setting
by Claire Jones-Manning

Music therapy is a non-invasive technique of distraction. As health care practitioners we strive to provide a holistic approach to patient treatment while enabling patients to be involved with the choice of care provided (Levine, 1971).

Sveto and Yung (1999) highlight that pre-operative anxiety is a common problem for theatre staff looking after patients. Waiting in a theatre holding area has been cited as anxiety provoking for patients (Kaempf and Amodei, 1989). Practitioners caring for anxious patients in the pre-operative phase are interested in evidence-based strategies on how to reduce psychological anxiety.

There is evidence of both psychological and physical changes pre-operatively due to increased anxiety levels (Kaempf and Amodei, 1989). Anxiety produces an imbalance in natural homeostasis (Green, 1996); physiologically, heart rate increases, blood pressure rises and there is an increase in palpitations. There is also evidence to suggest that components of the immune system are inhibited, provoking a greater susceptibility to post-operative infections (Green, 1996). A holistic approach to care needs to be found, using the knowledge that harm can be caused by increased stress levels. Strategies for reducing stress need to be found. Biley (1992) suggests that music therapy will reduce anxiety thus potentially reducing a hospital stay. Music, according to Biley (1992), has a bearing upon the holistic service we provide and needs further investigation. Allen (2001) found that listening to music pre-operatively reduces blood pressure and anxiety in patients. However, no further follow up studies have been conducted. The findings have a potentially huge impact for surgical patients.

The use of music therapy in the reduction of anxiety has been studied widely and is already utilized in some areas of patient care, such as intensive therapy units (Hancock, 1996) and also within theatre holding areas (Kaempf and Amodei, 1989).

The choice of music is very important. Patients should be given the opportunity to select music they can relate to (Stevens, 1990). Ethnicity also needs to be considered (Fischer, 1990). It is generally felt that tranquil relaxing music is more therapeutic across a range of ethnic backgrounds. Sveto and Yung (1999) looked at a small-scale group of Chinese patients and concluded that music can reduce anxiety in the anaesthetic room. Ethnicity was not an issue in this study.

Oliver (1999) states that music can create a warmer more pleasant environment for patients and staff and creates a diversion for patients. Hicks (1992) examined spinal anaesthesia and how the use of headsets can prevent overhearing inappropriate conversations.

Allen (2001) conducted research into a small group of patients with regard to blood pressure levels before surgery. She found patients had high blood pressure the morning before surgery, which she associated with high levels of stress and apprehension. Another reason suggested was that patients lose autonomy and this adds to their anxiety. Enabling patients to exert control by choosing which music to listen to may reduce stress by distraction and give them something personal to focus on. This was a small-scale study, however the author feels it can be used as a prelude to future research.

Kaempf and Amodei (1989) found that patients' anxiety levels decrease with the use of music. The conclusion from their study is that policies need to be developed to allow patients to use their own music within the operating room holding area.

The studies reviewed here were small scale with no clear picture of the benefit to the patient. However, they provide a good basis for further research.

Wigram et al (2002) quoting Ruud present four levels of music. The physiological level looks purely at the physiological effects and the medical potential of music, it was felt that this is the most useful level to look at for use within the anaesthetic room. It studies the physiological effects of music, mainly on heart rate, blood pressure and respiration.

Bruscia (1998) also explored basic properties of music and found the objective level directly influenced homeostasis, behaviour and anxiety levels, in an observable way.

Alvin (1975) states that we should never ignore the physical effect of music but draws no conclusion and offers no suggestion of what that music should be nor how it will affect the physiological status of the patient.

Music to reduce stress and anxiety should be without any major changes in tempo or pace (Winnicott, 1971). Bonny (1990) feels this should be with classical music but she shows a very limited view of music and does not accept patient choice. Saperston (1989) looked at the age of the patient and concluded that this had an effect on the type of music that will relax the patient. This again was a small-scale study that examined age, and no other factor was taken into consideration. This has not helped to gain an insight into what type of music will relax a patient within the anaesthetic room. Landreth et al (1974) found effects of music can be both stimulating and relaxing depending on the individual and the environment.

A psychological insight into music found that music can reduce anxiety and pain. Dileo (1993) describes the psychological level as supportive, reducing anxiety and pain, and acting as a distraction. It has certain characteristics, which are a medium, slow tempo with 60–80 beats per minutes (Bonny, 1990; Wigram, 2002). This is said to be a soothing rate by Moss (1988). However, no other variables were offered. Szeto and Yung (1999) concluded that soothing music should be played in the holding area of a theatre but offer no psychological or physical explanation for this.

Steady predictable rhythm, simple structure with recognizable melodies or themes, simple consonant harmony without sudden shifts or modulations, and stable dynamics without sudden shifts or contrasts are all considered important by Landreth and Landreth (1974). They found physical changes in a small group of patients when they played music with different rhythms. A steady rhythm relaxed the group. This study does not conclusively show evidence of the benefits of either predictable or unpredictable rhythm, structure or harmony.

Music cannot express emotions but rather creates moods to which we respond at an emotional level (Wigram et al, 2002). Music therapy will, if utilized to its full potential, help to create a peaceful environment. With education and evidence-based research the use of music as a complementary therapy can be harmoniously incorporated within the operating theatre.

Relaxation and imagery for pain control in children
by Sarah Roberts

This practice example aims to explore the use of relaxation and imagery as a means of helping children cope with pain and painful procedures. In order to do this it is necessary to explore the relationship between pain and anxiety and how the physical and emotional experiences of pain exist together. The techniques of relaxation and imagery will be discussed critically in relation to children in pain. Examples from the author's experience will be used to illustrate the use of these therapies in practice. The area of consent and professional accountability will also be explored in relation to children and their participation in their treatment.

Pain is a complicated concept to define due to its multi-factorial nature. The International Association for the Study of Pain (1979) defines it as

'An unpleasant sensory and emotional experience with actual or potential tissue damage or described in terms of such damage.'

It goes on to say,

'Pain is always subjective; each individual learns the application of the word through experiences related to injury in early life.'

The experience of pain is not just physical but is also affected by other sensory input (Melzack and Wall, 1982). Both these definitions recognize the effect of emotion on the experience of pain. Although this may seem obvious, conventional treatment does little to address this. Drugs may be given in an attempt to control pain physiologically but few nurses and doctors have had any formal training in how to address the emotional components of pain. This omission can have long-lasting effects on children who have been subject to painful conditions or procedures.

Anxiety is an emotion commonly associated with pain; it can be described as 'a fear of the unknown, as disproportionate to the treatment involved and directly related to future events in the life of the individual' (Swindale, 1989). This definition can be applied to children undergoing short-lived but nonetheless painful procedures, children in acute pain and children suffering chronic pain. Fear of the unknown associated with pain has been demonstrated countless times in my experience when children are unable to fully understand what is happening and do not know when the pain will stop. Children may also view the pain as a punishment for previous actions, and, particularly when injured doing something they knew to be wrong, this can cause further anxiety. The involvement of the limbic system in pain perception is thought to be the root of the feelings of anxiety and stress associated with pain (Moriarty, 1998; Carter, 1994).There is a growing body of evidence that suggests stress and anxiety can have a detrimental effect on the health and well-being of an individual (Friedman et al, 1969; Selye, 1976; Cohen and Williamson, 1991; McGrath, 1993).

All children subjected to pain, whatever the cause, will suffer some anxiety, fear and sadness related to their experience. It has been shown there is a positive relationship between anxiety levels and pain perception (Brugal, 1971). Pain or the anticipation of pain is seen as a threat by most humans and this causes activation of the sympathetic nervous system. This results in physical changes known as the 'fight or flight response', characterized by an increase in heart rate, blood pressure, respiratory rate, acuity of the senses, blood flow to voluntary muscles, blood glucose and sweat gland activity (Payne, 2000). Relaxation can help to calm this response by increasing the activity of the parasympathetic nervous system which reverses these changes (Benson, 1976).

The emotional distress of parents can exacerbate a child's anxiety and subsequently increase that child's experience of pain. This has been found to be particularly true in my experience when dealing with children who have potentially life-limiting conditions and also in children with horrific injuries. Parents require emotional and psychological support and realistic reassurance in order to support their children when they are in pain (McGrath, 1993). As health professionals we should aim to support all the physical and emotional needs of both the child and the family when treating pain. We should work in partnership with the child and family, giving control of the event to the child and providing internal mechanisms that suppress pain perception (Jonas et al, 1998).

The ideas of using relaxation, imagery and visualization in heath care are not new. States of induced trance have been used in healing throughout the centuries in many different cultures and countries, with China, Egypt, North America, Greece, Africa and Britain being examples (Rankin-Box, 1995). Relaxation can be described as 'a state of consciousness characterized by feelings and release from tension, anxiety and fear', and visualization as 'using the imagination to create desired changes in an individual's life' (Rankin-Box, 2001). Relaxation provides a reduction in anxiety and muscle tension and can increase a person's tolerance to pain and ability to cope with painful procedures (Carter, 1994).This reduction in muscle tension can have great benefits to the child in pain as holding muscles tense can in itself produce pain. This can be seen in children with abdominal pain who will often tense their abdominal muscles to protect the underlying organs. The consequence of this is they suffer pain not only from the organs but also from the tension in the muscles above them. Children who are faced with stressful situations either at home or at school may complain of headaches which are often caused by muscle tension in the neck. Relaxation does not reduce the intensity of the pain but it can reduce the distress associated with pain (McCaffery and Wong, 1993). I have found this to be true on many occasions when, after participating in a relaxation session, children report that although they still have their pain it does not bother them so much any more.

When dealing with children in pain the technique of guided imagery can be employed to facilitate relaxation and give children control to manage their pain. It is suggested that the use of imagination can be used to help children cope with frightening situations (Ott, 1996). Guided imagery involves children being guided through an image of their choice by a facilitator who asks questions such as, 'What can you see?', 'What can you smell?', 'How does it feel?', etc. The facilitator's questions are guided by the child's response. This has been described as 'engaging the child's imagination and concentration on a specific event to modify a particular response' (Doody et al, 1991). This technique can be used to provide distraction and pain relief for children undergoing procedures as well as those suffering more lasting pain. The facilitator should engage the child and attempt to win his or her trust for the imagery to be successful.

Ideally the child should be in as comfortable a position as possible in an environment with a comfortable temperature and free from distractions; this is often difficult to achieve in the hospital setting. The child should be encouraged to choose an image in which he or she would like to participate. As long as the child feels in control, the image can be anything, not necessarily something that adults may find relaxing; in my experience these images range from a trip to Sydney Opera House to a game of rugby. Once the image is chosen the child is encouraged to relax by whatever method works for him or her; this may take practice and some trial and error. Many techniques are described in the book *Relaxation Techniques: A practical handbook for health professionals* (Payne, 2000). I have found that most children like to image a warm feeling spreading up their body which makes them feel safe and relaxed. Once the child is relaxed the imagery begins. The duration of the session depends on the reactions of the child and also the reason for using imagery, e.g. for management of a procedure, the image must last for its entire duration.

There are various studies to support the use of imagery and relaxation in children with various health needs. Lai and Olness (1996) studied the effects of self-induced mental imagery in 76 children and found that all children showed a significant decrease in pulse rate and an increase in skin temperature during relaxing imagery. However, when the children took part in active imagery their pulse rate increased and electrodermal activity decreased. This study, although not clinically significant, does show the power of imagery to alter physiological functioning. It would also suggest that children should be encouraged to choose relaxing rather than active images. I have found, however, that as long as children can become involved in their image they gain benefit from it in the form of relaxation and a reduction of pain, whether they choose an active or a passive image. Broome et al (1994) studied the use of relaxation and imagery to reduce pain, parental anxiety and stress in children undergoing treatment for cancer. They demonstrated benefits to both children and their parents. However, the parents' and children's ability to use the techniques was not assessed. The effect of hypnosis and imagery on post-operative pain has been subject to a randomized controlled study. The results showed that although the use of analgesic medication did not alter between the experimental and control groups, the experimental group rated their pain significantly lower and their average hospital stay was shorter than the controls (Lambert, 1996). All these results are supported by Olness and Kohen (1996) who suggest that the benefits of using imagery and hypnosis as pain relief are:

- Reduction in anxiety.
- Enhancement of mastery and hope.
- Increased co-operation.
- Reduction in anxiety for family and health care professionals.

As previously mentioned I have noted these benefits on numerous occasions when caring for children and their families.

Relaxation and imagery techniques are not always suitable for all children. The cognitive ability of the child must be considered before imagery is undertaken. It has been suggested that children need to have reached Piaget's pre-operational stage (age 2–7 years) to benefit from guided imagery as a pain control therapy (Whitaker and McArthur, 1998). It is also argued that until the child reaches 8 or 9 years of age guided imagery with a facilitator is the only type of imagery that will succeed in obtaining benefit for the child (McGrath and Craig, 1989; Hobbs et al, 1980). Facilitators must be aware of child protection procedures and not allow themselves to be placed in a compromising position. Having a parent or another member staff in the room should avoid this. If a child discloses abuse during an imagery session the image should be swiftly drawn to a close and the situation dealt with according to the institution's usual child protection procedures.

Children need to be actively involved in the imagery and both they and their parents must have given informed consent to participating in the imagery as well as any procedure they are to undergo. The Nursing and Midwifery Council (2002) states that consent must be gained before any treatment or care can be carried out. This is to prevent infringement of the patient's autonomy. Indeed the UKCC (2000) states that all care procedures should be undertaken within a 'framework of informed consent'. In order for the child and family to give informed consent they require information and explanations they are able to understand. It is therefore important that the practitioner is skilled and knowledgeable in the techniques of facilitating relaxation and imagery. Various short courses exist for nurses to gain these skills, however as yet no course has been validated by nursing regulatory bodies. This can lead to potential problems as all nurses may not be taught to the same standards or by the same methods. Until validated courses are available the use of relaxation and imagery will be limited to those individuals who are interested in the subject and have taken steps to educate themselves.

The Nursing and Midwifery Council (2000) in the Code of Professional Conduct states,

> *'You must ensure that the use of complementary or alternative therapies is safe and in the interests of patients and clients. This must be discussed with the team as part of the therapeutic process and the patient or client must consent to their use.'*

This is paramount when dealing with children in pain and the use of relaxation and/or imagery should be offered as a package of care alongside conventional methods of providing analgesia.

The use of relaxation and imagery with children in pain can be a useful adjunct to conventional treatments. As discussed, there are studies that support its use with children and families to provide distraction and reduction in anxiety. In my experience children are very receptive to using these techniques, possibly due to their active imaginations. More studies are required to enable these techniques to become an accepted part of normal treatment for children in pain because, like many complementary therapies, much of the supporting evidence available is anecdotal. As has been demonstrated it is widely accepted that pain causes anxiety and yet conventional treatments do little to address this. If we as health care professionals do not provide methods that allow children in pain to take control and manage their anxiety we are doing them a great disservice. It could be argued that by not addressing the emotional aspects of pain control we are contravening the Human Rights Act (1998) that states,

> *'No one shall be subjected to torture or to inhumane or degrading treatment or punishment.'*

Relaxation and imagery are techniques that, if used appropriately, can help ensure that all aspects of a child's experience of pain are addressed.

References

Allen K (2001) Music reduces surgery stress. *BBC News* 25 May.

Alvin J (1975) *Music Therapy*. London. John Claire Books

Benson H (1976) *The Relaxation Response*. London: Collins.

Biley F (1992) Using music in hospital settings. *Nursing Standard* **6**(35): 37–9.

Bonny H (1990) Music and change. *Journal of the New Zealand Society for Music Therapy*. **12**(3): 5–10.

Broome ME, Lillis PP, McGahee TW, Bates T (1994) The use of distraction and imagery with children during painful procedures. *Eur J Cancer Care* **3**: 26–30.

Brugal MA (1971) Relationships of pre-operative anxiety and post-operative pain. *Nursing Research* **20**(1): 26–31.

Bruscia KE (1998) *Defining Music Therapy* (2nd edn). Gilson NH: Barcelona Publishers.

Carter B (1994) *Child and Infant Pain: Principles of Nursing Care and Management*. London: Chapman and Hall.

Cashell L, Miner A (1983) Role conflict and ambiguity among creative art therapists. *The Arts in Psychotherapy* **10**: 93–8.

Cohen S, Williamson GM (1991) Stress and infectious disease in humans. *Psychology Bulletin* **109**(1): 5–24.

Dalley T (1984) *Arts as a Therapy: An introduction to the use of art as a therapeutic technique*. New York: Routledge.

Dileo C (1993) *Music Therapy: International Perspective*. Pennsylvania: Jeffery Books.

Doody SB et al (1991) Non-pharmalogical intervention for pain management. *Critical Care Nursing Clinics of North America* **3**(1): 69–75.

Fischer M (1990) Music as therapy. *Nursing Times* **86**(38) 39–41.

Friedman SB, Glasgow LA, Ader R (1969) Psychological factors modifying host resistance to experimental infections. *Ann NY Acad Sci* **164**: 381–93.

Green KS (1996) Can music therapy reduces anxiety in theatre? *British Journal of Theatre Nurses* **5**(11): 24–7.

Hancock H (1996) Implementing change in management of postoperative pain. *Intensive Critical Care Nursing* **11**: 359–62

Heywood K (2002) Introducing art and therapy into the Christie Hospital, Manchester. *Complementary Therapies in Nursing and Midwifery* **9**: 125–32.

Hicks F (1992) The power of music. *Nursing Times* **88**(41): 72–4.

Hobbs SA, Moguin LE, Tyroler M, Lahey BB (1980) Cognitive behaviour therapy with children: Has clinical utility been demonstrated? *Psych Bull* **87**: 147–65.

International Association for the Study of Pain (1979) *Child and Infant Pain: Principles of Nursing Care*. London: Chapman and Hall.

Johnson G (2000) Should nurses practise complementary therapies? *Complementary Therapies in Nursing and Midwifery* **6**: 120–3.

Kaempf G, Amodei ME (1989) The effect of music on anxiety. *American Operating Room Nurses Journal* **50**(1): 112–18.

Kearney M (2000) *A Place of Healing*. New York:Oxford University Press.

Lai L, Olness K (1996) Effects of self-induced mental imagery and autonomic reactivity in children. *Developmental and Behavioural Paediatrics* **17**(5): 323–7.

Lambert SA (1996) The effects of hypnosis/guided imagery on the post-operative course of children. *Journal of Developmental and Behavioural Paediatrics* **17**(5): 307–10.

Landreth J, Landreth J (1974) Effects of music on physiological response. *Journal of Research in Music Education* **22:** 4–12

Levine ME (1971) Holistic nursing. *Nursing Clinics of North America* **6**: 253.

McCaffery M, Wong D (1993) Nursing interventions for pain control in children. In Schecter NL, Berde CB, Yaster M (eds) *Pain in Infants, Children and Adolescents*. Baltimore, MA: Williams and Wilkins.

McGrath PJ (1993) Psychological aspects of pain perception. In Schecter NL, Berde CB, Yaster M (eds) *Pain in Infants, Children and Adolescents*. Baltimore, MA: Williams and Wilkins.

McGrath PJ, Craig KD (1989) Developmental and psychological factors in pediatric pain. *Pediatric Clinics of North America* **36**: 823–36.

Melzack R, Wall P (1982) *The Challenge of Pain*. Harmondsworth: Penguin Books.

Moriarty A (1998) *Paediatric Pain Management. A multidisciplinary approach*. Oxford: Radcliffe Medical Press.

Moss A (1988) Music and the surgical patient: The effect of music on anxiety. *American Operating Room Nurses Journal* **48**(1): 64–9.

Nursing and Midwifery Council (2000) *Nursing Competencies*. London: Nursing and Midwifery Council.

Oliver J (1999) Music in theatres. *British Journal of Theatre Nurses* **9**(10): 460–3.

Olness K, Kohen D (1996) *Hypnosis and Hypnotherapy with Children*. London: Guilford Press.

Ott MJ (1996) Imagine the possibilities. Guided imagery with toddlers and pre-schoolers. *Pediatric Nursing* **22**(1): 34–8.

Payne R (2000) *Relaxation Techniques, A Practical Handbook for the Health Care Professional*. Edinburgh: Churchill Livingstone.

Rankin-Box D (ed) (1995) *The Nurses' Book of Complementary Therapies* (Revised edn) Edinburgh: Churchill Livingstone.

Rankin-Box D (ed) (2001) *The Nurses' Book of Complementary Therapies* (2nd edn). London: Bailliere Tindall.

Russell-Lacey S (1979) An experimental study of pictures produced by acute schizophrenic subjects. *Br J Psychiatry* **134**: 195–200.

Saperston B (1989) Music-based individualised relaxation training. A stress reduction approach for the behaviourally disturbed mentally retarded. *Music Therapy Perception* **6**: 26–33.

Schaverien J (1999) *The Revealing Image*. London: Jessica Kingsley Publishers.

Selye H (1976) The stress of life. In Rankin-Box D (ed) *The Nurses' Book of Complementary Therapies* (2nd edn). London: Bailliere Tindall.

Stevens K (1990) Patients' perceptions of music during surgery. *Journal of Advanced Nursing* **15:** 1045–51.

Swindale JE (1989) The nurse's role in giving pre-operative information to reduce anxiety in patients admitted to hospital for elective minor surgery. *Journal of Advanced Nursing* **14**(11): 899–905.

Sveto CK, Yung P (1999) Introducing music programme to reduce preoperative anxiety. *British Journal of Theatre Nurses* **9**(10): 455–9.

Teasdale C (1988) *Conditions of Service of Art Therapists*. London: MSF.

Thomson M (1997) *On Art and Therapy: An Exploration*. New York: Virago Press.

Waller D (1993) *Group Interactive Art Therapy: Its Use in Training and Treatment*. New York: Routledge.

Waller D, Gilroy A (1992) *Art Therapy: A Handbook*. Buckingham: Open University Press.

Warren B (1993) *Using Creative Arts in Therapy: A Practical Introduction*. New York: Routledge.

Whitaker B, McArthur L (1998) *Course notes. Relaxation and Guided Imagery. A Paediatric Pain Intervention for Health Professionals*. Liverpool: Royal Liverpool Children's Hospital NHS Trust.

Wigram T, Pedersen I, Bonde L (2002) *A Comprehensive Guide to Music Therapy* (p 58). London: Jessica Kingsley Publishers.

Winnicott D (1971) *Playing and Reality*. New York: Basic Books.

Index

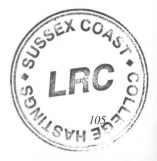